MAGIC AT OAKWELL

Discovering Herbal Healing

Phyllis Heitkamp M.H.

authorHOUSE®

AuthorHouse™
1663 Liberty Drive
Bloomington, IN 47403
www.authorhouse.com
Phone: 1-800-839-8640

First published by AuthorHouse   8/31/2009

ISBN: 978-1-4389-9976-0 (sc)

Printed in the United States of America
Bloomington, Indiana

This book is printed on acid-free paper.

Disclaimer

This book was written to assist you in making decisions regarding your health care. We need to be a part of the decision-making process in regard to our health. As you learn what is available, you can assist your health care provider and take responsibility for your part. Always find a health care provider that encompasses your philosophy of health and work together. It is your body and you need to make the final decision but this is impossible unless you find all of your options. This book is just one of many options that you have, find as many as you can before you make your "informed" decision.

Dedication and Memory

This book is dedicated to my loving and patient husband, LaVern Heitkamp.

I want to thank my son, Loren Paul Grayson for his encouragement to write my memories and philosophies that took the form of my Maggie Browne blogs.

This book couldn't have been written without the help of Linda Pavlovich, my first herbal student and her encouragement to continue to teach about herbs.

Bernard Rosen has contributed to my knowledge of nutrition and kept me updated on what is happening in the world of alternative medicine.

Letitia Read and Marie Calarco need to be thanked for their guidance in the editing of these writings.

Elizabeth Beasley is the creative genius that formulated the cover of this book.

In addition to the above I need to acknowledge:

Betty Westphal, Rebecca Noble, Marc and Heidi Lemke, Fran Kingery, Beth Passons, Gloria Hitzler, Susan Denzer, Kathy Grayson, Blaine Grayson, Carol Harris, Dorothy Dyken, Annie Gray and many more whose names should be here.

I would like to acknowledge the "Girls" that encouraged this to go forward:

Marie Calarco, Sue Robbins, Bonnie Beeck, and Linda Pavlovich

This book is in memory of Donna Lemke and Catharine Harris

Foreword

Bernard Rosen, PhD   February 2009

These are interesting times that we live in today. Everything happens so fast. There are new discoveries all the time. Claims of what is new and best. Before you know it the latest and greatest is all over the Internet and everyone in the free world is linked in. As a nutrition consultant and educator, I've come to realize one eternal truth. What's new and best isn't always the answer. In fact, it is often the opposite. What's tried and true, the wisdom of the generations; that is the ultimate truth. I'm a big believer in nature. Or as I say to my clients, "What do you think is more likely to be right? How something exists in nature or what man/woman has done to it?" In these terms the answer is quite clear.

One of the results of this fast pace is that we tend to get ahead of ourselves and not think things through real clearly. We take action because "someone" determined that "something" had to be done. Not necessarily the right thing, but something. So while at this time we are seeing states adopt Health Freedom Bills encouraging free choice for health care, we are seeing these same states adopt laws restricting our choices, and seeing practitioners argue over who is licensed, certified, and who has the right to practice. In the area of nutrition over 30 states currently have laws telling us who can give nutritional advice and who cannot, without any connection to whether or not their advice is sound or health giving.

We are faced with the threat of more regulations at all levels of government. On the International scene we have Codex, which threatens to let other countries dictate what we do here in the United States. If implemented, therapeutic dosages of herbs, supplements, vitamins and minerals will ultimately become unavailable as they will become illegal through the mechanisms that Codex puts in place. Natural health practitioners will be without their key instrument to help people while at the same time health conscious people will lose their choices for natural options. At the federal level we see more and more government involvement in health care. That means the government is telling you what you can and cannot do, who can get treatment and who cannot.

With our choices becoming limited we need to take responsibility for our own health. Being ill is expensive and your treatment may not be within your control. The best way to help yourself is to stay healthy and live a healthy lifestyle. Learn to heal yourself.

Herbs are great because they are food. They are nutrition. They work because they give our bodies the nutrients that they are not getting otherwise. They allow us to heal ourselves. This is a book filled with timeless wisdom. The tried and true – the ultimate truth. This book is a gift for you. You can use this information now or any time in the future. You just need a little space in your back yard. It will work. Thank you Phyllis for sharing your knowledge with us.

Bernard Rosen, PhD is a Nutrition Consultant and Educator. He works with individuals, groups, and at corporations to create individualized nutrition and wellness programs. He is an expert in the field of Nutrition and Erectile Dysfunction. His office is in Thiensville, WI. To learn more, e-mail bernie@brwellness.com, or go to http://www.brwellness.com and http://brwellness.blogspot. com.

Linda Pavlovich R. N.

When I signed up for Phyllis' herbal classes I was looking for information to incorporate herbs into my diet. I did not realize what an affect it would have on my life.

I started using herbs on my four legged family members besides myself. I have used herbs on my dog when he would occasionally eat nonfood items and get constipated. A few herbs mixed together into suppositories which the dog ended up eating as treats helped move things along. You cannot force an 89 pound muscular dog to do anything he doesn't want to do.

One of my cats who was eight years old when adopted came with crystals in his urine and had frequent urinary tract infections. After numerous uses of various antibiotics and different foods I tried a combination of herbs made into a tea, a few drops on his food every day cleaned things up. Now I only use it occasionally for prevention.

One of my dogs sprained his leg on a Sunday afternoon and came limping into the house. Once inside he would not place any weight on that limb. I gathered some leaves from the garden and made a tea. Then I took a clean cloth and moistened it with the cooled tea and wrapped his limb. I kept rewetting the cloth and reapplied it all afternoon. By evening he was placing some weight on it and limping around. Within 48 hours he was running around like it had never happened.

The time of integrated medicine (alternative), Holistic and western methods is not only here for people but for our animals.

Today it is much easier to find a vet who uses herbs and other holistic methods or is at least open to discussing them with you. When talking with a master herbalist, know that your information is coming from a reliable source before discussing it with your vet.

Make sure to check with your vet on dosages as our pets weight a lot less than the average adult, (See chapter on Marshmallow for pet dosages.) Phyllis' books are not only interesting reading but great resource and reference material.

Our pets have dis-eases that sound a lot like our diseases that is because they are affected by the food and water that they consume, the stress around them and lack of exercise and fresh air.

One thing you can do right now is become a label reader. Can you pronounce the words, let alone know what they are? Are these preservatives, fillers, additives, or dyes in the food?

With so many foods available today you have more choices to clean up your pet's diet and still stay within your budget.

Pets also are feeling our stress, so the better we take care of ourselves the better we can take care of them. It is a win-win situation.

We can start by making some room in our yards for a few herbs. Make sure that they do not get pesticides on them as you will be eating them. You will be helping yourself and your pets.

Linda Pavlovich
RN. / Reiki Master
Animal Communicator
Animal Energy Work and Massages
Distance Energy Work and Animal Communication
262-251-9114

Introduction

I have wanted to write this book and talk about all the ways to co-create with plants. I wrote it in two parts, the first part being articles about plants that have so many abilities to heal humans. I should take that back as I know that herbs really don't heal bodies but give of themselves to our bodies for that purpose. First, they have the ability to give the lacking nourishment that each body craves and secondly, they give of themselves freely with love.

Each plant that I have worked with has the ability to connect with all the parts of anyone using it. Sometimes it amazes me that we attribute certain plants for certain things. The more lacking one is, the more that any plant will be of assistance. Plants do try to assist in one or more areas but have many abilities. If they need something to do a job, they will draw what they need to them.

We have learned to eat on schedules for our life styles, yet people who are healthy, are ones who are not on a schedule but eat when their body tells them that it would be a good idea.

Gardeners are most fortunate in this regard as they have the availability to nibble on this or that while in their gardens. The unfortunate part of this is that most present-time gardeners do not avail themselves of this because they lack the knowledge; the intuition to feel comfortable doing this. Most gardeners see only the fruit of the plant and think that is all a plant has to offer. We wait months for the raspberries without knowing that nibbling on a leaf has so much for us. We pull weeds out from around the tomatoes and dump them in the recycling bin, thinking that we are doing a wonderful thing by cleaning the garden up and putting the refuse back into our soil; when these weeds are loaded with all sorts of minerals that could be used to rebuild our bodies.

It is my hope that as each person learns what is living around them, they will also learn to appreciate the gifts that nature supplies.

Sometimes I see a yard loaded with dandelions and I think to myself, someone in the dwelling needs help with their liver and here is their medicine. I know that if I walked into that house I would find people with high blood pressure or high cholesterol. Present-time people do not understand that nature knows more about us than we do about them.

In the second part of this book, I want to introduce a different way of looking at nature. Maybe there is someone who will pick up this book and says, "I knew there was more than what I was looking at."

We are all introduced to the spiritual side of nature as we can deal with it. We have been so distant from that idea for much too long. Nature waits and waits for us to wake up and communicate so that we can co-create on this planet.

At first nature reaches out to us with feelings as you will read about. They like to "worm" their way into our hearts and our whole being. We start as children marveling at each thing that nature presents to us and somewhere along the way, we lose this wondrous feeling. It must be sad to watch humans retreat from the world around them.

When do you think it happens? Are we so overwhelmed by learning the three Rs that nature takes a back seat? Have we become so civilized that we don't respond to the cries of nature as we butcher a plant or take the bounty without thanking each plant for it?

I hope that while reading about my experiences with these herbs and nature, it excites one person to step across the line into another world with me, the world of plants.

Herbally,
Phyllis Heitkamp

Table of Contents

Disclaimer..v
Dedication and Memory......................................vi
Foreword by Bernie Rosen and Linda Pavlovich.........vii
Introduction...xi

Part One

    Apple 3
    Barberry..7
    Bergamot...10
    Black Cohosh 12
    Black Walnut..14
    Blue Cohosh 17
    Blue Vervain 20
    Burdock 22
    Calendula 25
    Cascara Sagrada...28
    Catnip 30
    Cayenne 33
    Chamomile 37
    Chickweed 40
    Comfrey 43
    Dandelion 47
    Echinacea 51
    Fenugreek 54
    Feverfew..57
    Garlic 59
    Ginseng 62
    Hawthorn 64
    Horsetail Grass..68
    Hyssop...70
    Lamb's Quarters 72
    Marshmallow 74
    Lemon Balm 78
    Motherwort...81

Mullein 83

Oak 86

Peppermint 89

Plantain...92

Purslane 96

Queen Anne's Lace 98

Red Clover...100

Red Raspberry 102

Roses 105

Rosemary 107

Sassafras...110

Shepherd's Purse 113

Slippery Elm 115

St. John'swort 118

Stevia..121

Stinging Nettle 123

Strawberries 127

Wild Violets...129

Wood Betony 132

Wormwood...134

Yarrow...136

Yellow Dock 139

References 142

Index..144

Part Two

The World of Spirit...151

Co-creating with Plants..................................163

Feelings 167

The Apple Garden 171

Trees that Heal 174

The Others...176

We Are All One 182

The Magic of Life 185

The Seed as Physician...................................189

Insects are Friends 194

Dowsing...198

A Shaman 202
Hanna's Magic 205
Little Beings 210
Planet of Choice 213
Leap of Faith...217
Resources 219

Part One

Apple

Pyrus malus

Apple is a medicinal plant that grows just about everywhere. There are many varieties but they all contain the same medicinal properties.

When I was looking for some land to grow herbs, I told the gentleman that was helping me that I needed land that hadn't been chemically sprayed or fertilized for at least five years. We got into a discussion about medicinal herbs and the fact that it takes five years for the residue of chemicals to dissipate. Then when I use the plants to make medicine, I have no chemicals added to my formulas.

As we talked he asked if I could help him. He was unable to sleep at night in a bed. When he would lie down, his stomach acid would come up into his throat. For years he had slept in a reclining chair and still had the problem.

I suggested one tablespoon of organic apple cider vinegar in 6 to 8 ounces of water, to be sipped on, one hour before he went to bed. When mentioning apple cider vinegar, I don't mean the processed kind. We want the kind that isn't clear and has some "mother" in it. According to Jethro Kloss, author of BACK TO EDEN, "The ordinary apple cider is not fit to be used." But if you have the clear white processed kind, use it to clean windows and flower vases as it will dissolve the minerals on glass very well. The Organic Apple Cider Vinegar with some of the apple settled on the bottom of the jar will dissolve the minerals that are in the body that are being parked in the joints creating arthritis and along the arteries, creating a hardening effect.

3

According to Dr. Christopher, founder of the School of Natural Healing; most of us have gotten into the habit of not chewing our foods when we eat. He suggests that we "Drink our food and chew our liquids." This means chewing or mixing the saliva with our drinks as well as our food. This is the first step in digestion. It is also the first step in health as saliva will decrease the in-take of germs.

Germs have a very narrow range of pH. Saliva is alkaline and will kill the germs not happy in that environment. The stomach has an acid environment so the germs not liking that pH will be killed. By mixing the saliva with your food, you have gotten rid of probable 40% of germs that you are taking in. Germs have a job and they are everywhere. We need to learn to live with them or in this case, around them.

What usually happens is that we make the stomach do all the work and by the time we are 40 or 50 years old, our stomach has the "acid making valves" set ON all the time. What do you think happens when we take an antacid? Right, it temporarily helps but then the stomach needs to get back to its natural state, which is acid, so it increases the amount of acid.

By sipping apple cider vinegar diluted in water, the stomach, getting a mild acid, recognizes this and stops producing more. (Yes, our bodies are that smart!)

A couple of days after suggesting the remedy to this man, I got a call from him thanking me for the best sleep he has had in years.

This is just one of the things Apples can do.

Hanna Kroeger, National Herbalist, talked about using Apple Peel Tea to pull toxins out of the body. I cut my organic apples peelings about 1/2 inch or more thick, dried these so when I wanted to use this tea, I boiled these peelings and served the tea that they make. (Children who want to taste my herbs are allowed to chew on these dried peelings. They tell me that my herbs are great.)

My Uncle Clarence told me how to keep the worms out of organic apples. Make a mixture of 50% vinegar and 50% honey. Put a little of this mixture in a wide-mouth jar and tape it to an almost horizontal branch of the apple tree just as the flower buds start coming out. Leave them on until the last petal falls off. You will have to clean the bugs out of the mixture several times, but they will not be laying eggs in the flowers, hence your new apples.

Kloss called Apples the "King of Fruits." He suggested that people who have too much acid, eat sweet apples and those with not enough acid should eat sour-green apples.

Even the very old and the very young do well on scraped apples. Kroeger suggested that "Whatever ails you; gall bladder trouble, liver trouble, diarrhea, tooth decay, constipation, loss of appetite, (even) good as poultices, too. When someone is very ill, take an apple and scrape the meat with a silver spoon. You will see them get better."

Kroeger was "big" on silver. She said that silver kills germs. When you toss a silver coin in the well, the whole village stays healthy. (They are on their own for the happiness part.) I do not recommend Colloidal Silver for anyone. When you take silver into the body in large amounts, it is the same as taking a medical antibiotic. It kills off the good flora in the small intestines. Eating off a silver spoon will put silver into the body and the food that carries it but will not destroy the flora. According to Kroeger, silver also repels negative forces. I suggest that people wear this on their person.

Apple pectin is found to clean the bowels and has been put into many herbal formulas.

Dr. Christopher's *Super Garlic Immune Formula* is a formula that I have used with success to handle major problems. It contains: Garlic, Lobelia, Marshmallow Root, White Oak Bark, Black Walnut, Mullein, Aloe Vera, Gravel Rt., Skullcap, Plantain, Apple Cider Vinegar, and Raw Honey.

My daughter called and told me that she had been ill for a week and was not getting better. I took my herbs to her house, when I got there I decided to give her the *Super Garlic Immune Formula*. I gave her a tablespoonful every hour for three hours. Her fever broke and she slept, waking up feeling fine. This formula did the trick.

Herbs can be taken every hour when working on a problem. We are talking about food. Herbs feed the body what it needs to

5

rebuild or get healthy. This is so contrary to what we have been taught about medicine. With chemical medicine, one can overdose but can one have too much pumpkin pie? I guess one could but it isn't dangerous just uncomfortable.

For more information on Garlic and how it works, go to my article on it.

Apple bark is very rich in oxygen, potassium, sodium, magnesium and iron.

Kloss mentioned that apple tree bark is an old fashioned remedy for fever and as a tonic. When taken hot it causes perspiration. This helps with the liver, spleen, kidneys, boils, insect bites, toothaches, and digestion.

You have probably heard about "Food combinations" to increase our energy. This is when you combine some foods with one group of foods but not with another group. Example: Bread goes well with fruit but not as well with meats. (What do we eat for lunch but meat sandwiches and wonder why we have no energy in the afternoon?) According to Kroeger, apples go with anything you wish to combine with them. For more information on food groups, see Hanna Kroeger's book THE BASIC CAUSES OF MODERN DISEASE AND HOW TO REMEDY THEM.

"An Apple a day keeps the doctor away" – has new meaning after looking at all it can do. Enjoy Apples in any form.

Barberry

Berberis vulgaris

What do I know about Barberry? I know that I have four of them in my yard. Two of these have dark purple leaves and two of them have yellow leaves.

I trim the yellow ones when they get straggly and my neighbors can't believe that I don't wear gloves when I do this. Barberry is one bush that is loaded with barbs; I supposed that is how she got her name? When I trim these ladies, I am referring to the yellow ones, I tell them that I am going to make they look attractive and everyone driving by will notice them. They really like that and allow me to cut the ends off without damage to either of us.

The two dark shrubs seem to stay in shape and rather small up near the house.

Okay, this is supposed to be about how they help medicinally and I have wandered into the Spiritual aspect of these plants. You will read more about that in Part Two of this book.

I checked with Dr. James Duke's database and thought that this would be a good place to tell you about some of the things that are in Barberry. I found 52 different constituents that allow them to do all the wonderful things they are capable of doing. I thought I would mention some that you might recognize starting with calcium, chromium, citric acid, iron, magnesium, manganese, niacin, phosphorus, potassium, protein, selenium, tin, and zinc.

Some of these were in very large amounts but well balanced with all the other things found in this wonderful plant. This is why I like Wholesome and not Part-some. When we take a capsule of just

7

calcium, all the balancing constituents are not there and we have really put this body out of balance. When we take some Barberry, all is in balance per God's design so we haven't put stress on our system.

What does it do with all of these things? Well, Barberry thinks that it can get out of the body through the liver. It heads for the liver. It is one of the best liver herbs around.

Dr. John R. Christopher always was talking about Berberis Vulgaris , he either liked that plant so much or he just liked saying Berberis Vulgaris. Either way it is one of the most important herbs for people to consider.

We mentioned that Barberry heads for the liver, so let's talk about the liver. Most of us think that our heart is the king of all our organs and we are wrong. The body depends on how healthy our liver is. The liver has so many jobs from making cholesterol that keeps our joints working and soft to detoxing every single chemical that is no longer needed in the body and getting it out in the form of gall.

Dr. Christopher was very adamant about NEVER EATING LIVER from any animal. The beef cow gets hooked on the barred fence and tears her hide. It festers and where does this toxic go? How about the chickens that are kept in confined areas? They get upset and take it out on the chicken next to them. The sores heal but the toxins go to the liver. And all these years your Grandmothers were insisting that you eat liver. Why? Because it is high in iron, but then so is Burdock, Dandelion and many other herbs.

It doesn't matter what you ingest, it is the liver that has to get rid of it. We are all eating more and more chemicals just because we are alive at this time in history. We have developed into a people who create chemicals for everything from cleaning to feeling well. We breathe these chemicals in from everywhere.

In our stressed out world, we create chemicals in our bodies just to try to deal with it all. When we are upset at the driver that cut in front of our car, we created a chemical that we feel from our toes to the tops of our heads. Where does this anger- chemical go? To the liver.

When we are in love, we are in love from the back of our eyeballs to the pit of our stomachs. This is another self developed chemical reaction that the liver has to deal with. I am not going to even mention hormones that the body creates.

Now let's add to this pot of chemicals that we are walking around with; how about an aspirin for the stress of driving in the same area as these weird people? Or maybe love has lost its luster and depression has set in, so let's take an antidepressant that Lily or Merck puts out? Look out liver here are more chemicals that need to be detoxed to keep this body healthy.

So what happens when we take some Barberry? Well, like all the rest it too heads for the liver too and with its 52 constituents, it helps the liver to release a lot of what it has been hanging on to. Yes, the liver does a lot of storage.

Barberry has a very bitter taste. According to an article that Dr. Duke wrote, "Bitter is better."

It is this bitter part that helps clean out the liver, a lot of the other constituents will stick around and help heal it. Hanna Kroeger, my mentor mentioned that if 10% of any organ is well, it can be rebuilt. I don't know if she was talking about the liver but she should have been.

What do organs need to rebuild? They need to have the building blocks to do this. When we give them what they need, they will service us for a very long time.

Barberry is just one of the many organs that we take for granted

Dr. Christopher said that a complete diet consists of: Fruits, Vegetables, Whole grains, Nuts and Seeds.

Bergamot

Monarda didyma

A couple of years ago I wanted a "Bee Balm" plant in my yard so one my friends gave me some of what she had in her yard. They were beautiful with their red tassels on the top of the plants. I put them in my back yard to add color. While riding my bike on the bike trail, I noticed these same plants growing wild along the sides of the trail only they had purple tassels on the top. So I did some investigating and found that wild Bee Balm or Bergamot is purple.

As I usually do, I "liberated" a few of these plants and put them in my yard. My usual habit is to wait until the plants go to seed and then take the seeds for my yard but these plants are so "nondescript" that I thought I might not recognize them without their purple tops. I was right. They are hard for me to sort out among all the weeds growing along the trail.

Then I set out to learn about them.

The first thing that I learned was that this whole plant is edible. I also have a book written by a Native American, Tis Mal Crow called NATIVE PLANTS, NATIVE HEALING -Traditional Muskogee Way. In this book Tis has a whole chapter devoted to this one plant, Wild Bergamot. If one is to believe this, the Muskogee tribe used this plant for everything, from lung infections, Tuberculosis, skin rashes, stings and bites, depression, anxiety, insomnia, burns, fevers, frostbite, scar tissue, digestion, blood Infections, ear Infections, sore muscles, Appendicitis, and even love potions. He mentioned that it is called Sweet Leaf and related to the mint family. When they make a tea out of this plant it is called OSWEGO TEA.

I went into Dr. Dukes Database to learn more. I could understand why the Native Americans could use this plant for everything. He has a list of about 60 different constituents in this plant and they were loaded with abilities to handle things like: bacteria, inflammation, Candida, Vermin, Virus and some even mentioned that they were antioxidant and anticancer along with being sedative.

We just don't give enough attention to things that our bodies could use that aren't found in the food or drug departments anywhere.

Black Cohosh

Cimicifuga racemosa

These plants grow wild all over in my area and it is a leaf that seems to be familiar but no one seems to be able to identify it in the wild. O.K. maybe it is just me. I was visiting my neighbor and mentioned that she had Black Cohosh growing in her yard. She told me that the plant was really Baneberry. I took a leaf off from her plant and brought it home to my Black Cohosh; it looked very close to the same leaf. (After a while you can't imagine all the leaf shapes that there are.) When mine flowered and put the tall spikes up, I took one over to her house, but her plants had fluffy feather-like flowers on a very short flat top. So they weren't the same plant even though they look alike.

So how do we know when we have a certain plant? I usually use a couple of identification books to help me do this and even when I can't find it in my books, I take a leaf off and put it into the book to be pressed and identified later. The books that I have found helpful are: PETERSON FIELD GUIDES – MEDICINAL PLANTS, and EYEWITNESS HANDBOOKS- HERBS. I like these two because they have drawings as well as pictures in them. I find that photos of plants don't give one all the characteristics to make a definite identification.

Black Cohosh made a big splash having to do with estrogen replacement for women who were in menopause. It seems that this herb was the buzz word for "I need help." I didn't understand that from an herbalist point of view because I could name fifteen to twenty herbs that are loaded with phyto-hormones. Black Cohosh is just one as are Catnip, Chamomile, Hops, Garlic, Raspberry leaves, Garden Sage and many more.

The problem is that most of the people talking about this herb are on some drug that is supposed to do this for them, like Pregnant Mare Urine, Premarin or some other medical drug high in estrogen. The high estrogen found in these drugs is detrimental to the body in regard to bone loss and even some thyroid problems.

The reason that I prefer one or more of the organic plants with estrogenic properties is that for the most part we don't need estrogen but by taking an herb with estrogenic properties, the body can decide what it needs and how much. It isn't given this choice with pills.

What the body really needs are herbs that give the body the phyto-hormones that allow the body to make what it needs to get and stay healthy. If the body needs more progesterone, the building blocks are available. If the body needs more testosterone, again the building blocks are there. The body is back in control and the symptoms lessen or stop all together.

According to The School of Natural Healing's director, David Christopher; for centuries women went through menopause without the help of a doctor. What we really need are minerals, vitamins and phyto-chemicals. With our present life style, we are not getting whole foods. There aren't any Black Cohosh farms. Wild plants have what we need and are not messed up with present time farming processes.

While discussing the need for vitamins, minerals and other health giving things in plants, Michael Pollan wrote in Omnivore's Dilemma, "You wonder what else is going on in these plants, what other undiscovered qualities in them we've evolved to depend on."

Black Cohosh is a wonderful plant. It is not only attractive and living in my yard but grows wild in my state. For those of you that still have trouble identifying it, then let me suggest that you head to the raspberry patch and make a tea out of raspberry leaves, or one of the other plants that I have mentioned in this article.

The School of Natural Healing suggests that by eating the proper diet of Whole Grains (loaded with phyto-hormones), Fruits, Vegetables, Nuts and Seeds, then your body will be getting what it needs to help you weather a lot of storms. Eat well and be well.

Black Walnut

Juglans nigra

Most people think of herbs as being little plants. I want to tell you about a very large one, the Black Walnut tree. Most people aren't happy having them growing in their yard because when the fruit falls, it makes a mess under the tree. The grass fights to grow under these large giants.

In spite of this, Black Walnut Tincture is my favorite herb. According to what I have read, Black Walnut has the ability to burn up excessive toxins and fat. It helps balance blood sugar in the body. It is Antiseptic and expels Parasites. That is a lot for one plant to be able to do. It is the high organic iodine in the hulls of the fruit that does a lot of this. Isn't it amazing that most plants that are high in organic iodine are found close to an ocean? Black Walnut is found thousands of miles from the nearest sea.

Dr. John R. Christopher, founder of the School of Natural Healing said, "Black Walnut Tincture is one of the best known remedies for fungus. Use it externally and apply frequently."

There is nothing written about it being Antiviral but I have witnessed it clearing warts from bodies. (A viral infection) My sister had warts all over her body so she was using this topically as well as internally on a daily basis. Within a short time (a few weeks) her warts fell off, right into the tub on toweling.

The iodine in Black Walnut is what is credited for a lot of its healing properties and I have used it to treat a thyroid deficiency conditions. Along with iodine, we find in a nutritional profile that this plant also contains high amounts of potassium, selenium, iron, magnesium and calcium. Dr. Christopher suggested getting more potassium into the family's diet by put some of the Black Walnut Tincture into soups or stews. The alcohol will dissipate with the heat of the food, leaving only the good stuff that you want to get into your food supply.

Hulda Clark author of THE CURE FOR ALL DISEASES suggests,"... take Black Walnut Tincture Extra Strength every week or until your illness is but a hazy memory. This is to kill any parasite stage you pick up from your family, friends or pets." This is not a bad idea and those of us who clean cat's litter boxes should take this to heart if we wish to stay healthy. That is not to say that we would do this every week but from time to time it is a very helpful thing to do.

As a dowser, there are times I tell people that the problem they are having is caused by parasites. Most people do not want to think that they are hosts to anything like this. The fact is that most of us host some parasites from time to time. How about the wonderful pet dog that you have who loves you so much that he licks your face. I know, you have him on heart worm medicine and he has been dewormed but we all share this planet, even parasites.

As a fungicide, Black Walnut Tincture is wonderful. My daughter used it topically on a toenail fungus. She also used it internally and in a month the fungus was cleaned up. When we use thing internally as well as externally, we are healing from the inside out and vice versa.

I had a peach tree that had peach tree fungus. So as an herbalist, I experimented. I took the end of one branch and put garlic oil on the leaves. I labeled that branch. The next branch that I worked on, I used the copper antifungal solution that I got for this from the garden shop. I labeled that branch. The next one that I worked on, I diluted my Black Walnut Tincture and put it all over those leaves. Then that one got labeled. After giving this project some time, I checked to see what was handling the problem. The Copper solution wasn't doing anything, the garlic solution wasn't either but the Black Walnut Tincture had cleaned up the end of its branch. So I diluted my Black Walnut Tincture 1 to 4 with water and sprayed the whole tree. It worked. But the solution killed the St. John's wort that was living under the tree. The next year I put a plastic drop cloth over my small plants under this tree before I sprayed.

Trees are amazing. If the Black Walnut tree runs out of what it needs to stay healthy, it puts out hair roots until it finds what is needed. This can be as deep as 50 to 75 feet below the surface of the ground. It really doesn't care what we do to the top few feet of ground (unless large amounts of chemicals are put there.)

This tincture can be used on cuts just like the old mercurochrome and it stings just like that did too.

Here are some interesting facts; tinctures get into the blood stream faster than herbal capsules do. They are carried there by the alcohol through the stomach wall and do not have to go through the digestive system. This makes them "fast-acting." Tinctures hold their healing properties for years. Dr. Christopher mentioned that he found some tinctures that were 40 years old and still did what he wanted them to do.

Blue Cohosh

Caulophyllum thalictroides

This lovely lady (and when you meet her you will feel the same as I do) is found in my Wisconsin woods. She has a fragile feeling about her. Her tulip-like leaves flutter eighteen to twenty-four inches off the floor of the forest. She prefers to be around mature trees where the leafy canopy is high over head, allowing small plants to thrive without much competition.

Her early flowers are in clusters and are hard to notice as they are greenish-yellow in color and blend in with the new foliage. By the time you notice Blue Cohosh; the "woodland spring flowers" have been in blossom awhile.

Blue Cohosh gets her name from the blue-green of her leaves and the bright blue berries that are found in the fall. Her common names are Squaw root, Papoose root, Blue Ginseng, and Yellow Ginseng, all of which you will understand as you read. Her leaves have three lobes ending almost the same length with the middle one sometimes having a two-toothed lobe. This gives the appearance of a blue-green tulip. I guess if I had been the one to name her, she would have been called the blue tulip plant.

The fruit of the flowers have "one or two seeds about the size of a large pea, which ripens in August," according to Mrs. Grieve in her A MODERN HERBAL, "these are sometimes roasted and boiled in water and given as a decoction resembling coffee." I like to replant these berries in woody areas

The roots are "hard thick, irregular, knotty contorted caudex (the base of the stem), one to several inches long, with slender

17

radicles (roots) up to 8 inches long, externally yellowy brown, internally whitish to yellow, with a central pith running longitudinally" all according to Mrs. Grieves.

As a medicinal herb, Blue Cohosh qualifies. It is said to have estrogenic properties. Historically it was prescribed by physicians for cramps and chronic uterine diseases.

A study in India suggests that the roots may possess some contraceptive properties.

Blue Cohosh has been used to relieve childbirth pains when given at the proper time, which means that it should only be taken in the last month of pregnancy.

Although I have called this plant a she and so far have discussed her uses for women, she is very helpful for men as well.

Blue Cohosh has been used successfully for rheumatism, epilepsy, leucorrhea, neuralgia, dropsy, hysteria, palpitations of the heart, high blood pressure and Diabetes. I have read that it is also good for hiccoughs and Whooping cough. A tea can be used for children with colic.

Jethro Kloss, author of BACK TO EDEN wrote, "Blue Cohosh contains the following vital minerals; potassium, magnesium, calcium, iron, silicon, and phosphorus. These minerals help to alkalize the blood and urine. This herb can be quite irritating to mucus surfaces and therefore should be used with some caution. It should not be used during pregnancy and should be taken only one week at a time, one to three capsules daily."

When I went to Dr. James A. Duke's database, I found a lot of things that this plant has the ability to work on. Here are just a few of the many: Antibacterial, Anticancer, Antidiabetic, AntiHIV, Antiinflammatory, Antioxidant, Antispasmodic, Candidicide, Cardioprotective, Pesticide, Vasoconstrictor and Vasodilator. These last two are a reminder that even when a plant works in one direction, it also has the ability to work in another direction. It is the plant working with the body that does the healing. The body knows what of this plant is needed and the plant supplies it.

It has been my experience that most people using this herb combine it with other herbs in making formulas. When we put together a formulation, we are looking for that formula to do a certain thing. We combine the herbs that will help us in this manner.

One of the formulas contains Blue Cohosh is Dr. John R. Christopher's B & B Tincture. This formulation is used as a nerve and hearing loss/ earache formula. Due to the formulation, it is great internally and externally. In this formula Dr. Christopher combines Blue Cohosh with four other nervine herbs. Dr. Christopher says that this formula can be "Used to aid in nervous conditions, sore throat, hiccups and restore malfunctioning motor nerves." The combination is designed to go to the nerves that are in trouble and help with the rebuilding. When my thumb muscles didn't work without hurting after my arm was taken out of a cast, I dropped B&B tincture on the skin and allowed it to be absorbed. When the nerves had been relaxed, I manually worked those muscles and in a short time, I was able to use the thumb without assistance and discomfort.

According to Dr. Christopher in his *Natural Healing Newsletter, Volume 5, no. 9,* "Dr. King of the Eclectic School of Medicine employed Blue Cohosh for its benefits on the mucous membranes. Later Dr. Scudder believed Blue Cohosh effected its good through the hypogastric plexus, thus affecting the circulation, nutrition, and reproduction."

Herbs are designed to cleanse and ***help the body rebuild.*** They supply the building blocks and allow the body to heal.

Blue Vervain

Verbena officinalis

I was teaching a class in my husband's hometown and one of his school classmates attended my classes. She was so excited about the class that she wanted to give me a plant. After the classes were done we went to her house near the lake and she dug up a Vervain for me. She told me that she never knows where they were going to grow until they come up because they tend to move around. (Plants have a way of doing this at my house too.)

This three foot plant didn't look much like anything until it put out its long fingered flower spikes. The flowers grow on these spikes coming out of the top of this plant. They are nice little blue/purple flowers that open a few at a time until they have all opened.

Vervain is said to handle kidneys stones, jaundice, stomach pains and much more.

Dr. James Duke's database mentions that there were a little over 20 constituents in this plant with many of them being very Antiinflammatory and Antiviral. This always means anticancer to me. It did have one property that was AntiHIV. So for a small plant, it contains some heavy duty stuff.

According to Richard Mabey in his book The NEW AGE HERBALIST, Vervain has been used mostly for liver and gall problems along with nerves and for depression. He also sees it as being good for promoting lactation and menses.

When was the last time that you fed your nerves? These are long cells and they tend to break down just like all of our other cells do on a daily basis. They need to be rebuilt, or replaced constantly.

Mabey talked about four plants that were good at doing this and Vervain was one of them, the other three were: Wild Oats, Ginseng, and Skullcap.

I read where the Romans used this plant to purify their homes and temples. So here we have some spiritual properties of this plant. In part two of this book, I want to talk a lot about the spiritual properties of plants.

Dr. Richard Bach, the father of flower remedies used it to handle stress and over- exertion. According to Joyce Petrak, DCH., in HOW TO REMEMBR BACH FLOWER REMEDIES...

She pointed out that Vervain was a very "upright perennial" and she equated this with a very positive outlook. "Many of the wrongs of the world have been righted by positive Vervains who calmly and wisely inspire other to noble causes."

As you have guessed, this will be the next tincture that I tackle for my medicine chest.

We all need to boost our nervous system from time to time so that we are ready for the next adventure that is ahead of us.

Burdock

Arctium lappa

Everything that I write about Burdock, like all that I write, is not just for Burdock Major but the Burdock plant that is growing in your back yard.

Most of us hate the burs that our pets bring into the house attached to their fur but it is the most successful way that this plant has of spreading its seeds. This is obvious as we find Burdock growing everywhere.

Right up front, Burdock root is a blood cleanser. Does that mean that it goes in and screens the blood system? No, it means that it forces the cells to release toxins into the blood to be cleaned from the system.

Burdock is such a wonderful blood cleanser that it is the main ingredient in Essiac. ESSIAC – A NATIVE HERBAL CANCER REMEDY by Cynthis Olsen tells the story of Essiac as a native herbal cancer remedy. The story goes that Native Americans in Canada couldn't believe what was being done for cancer. They mentioned this herbal combination to a nurse and she started using it on her patients with much success. She was only a nurse and ended up in court for practicing medicine without a license even though what she had done had helped hundreds of people to live a longer and cancer- free life. A Dr. Charles Brusch of Massachusetts came to her rescue and told the court that he would allow her to treat patients with this formula under his license. (This doctor, by the way become President John F. Kennedy's primary physician)

The formula was one that the nurse kept secret for a very long time and finally released it. The following is the combination:

6.5 cups – cut Burdock Root (52 measuring cup oz.)
16 oz - Powdered Sheep Sorrel
4 oz. - Powdered Slippery Elm
1 oz. – Turkey Rhubarb Root

When I read about the hundreds of people that she was able to help, even her mother was diagnosed with cancer and by giving her this combination in tea form, her mother lived for years without the disease. Many people testified on her behalf when she went to court but the law is inflexible. (Read the foreword by Rosen)

At one time she had a research laboratory do tests with the formula on mice and the researchers said that it didn't work on mice. It was then that she found the plants that were being used were frozen and decided to be careful who would get the formula. Finally prior to her death in 1978, she gave the formula to a Canadian company. This is just one wonderful story about Burdock but I tell it only because it talks about just how powerful this herb is.

In the orient, Burdock is used as a food and could be here in the United States. Burdock root has a rather mild taste and even after cooking only adds to whatever is being made. In Wisconsin there is a company in the middle of the state that harvests and sells fresh Burdock. When I want to have my students taste it, I purchase fresh root from the produce department of a health food store in Milwaukee. My students are amazed at the mild taste. It can be added to salads or anything that one is eating.

The purpose of my class is to show my students how to use herbs in different ways. They read all the books on what is good for what but even if it is growing in their backyards they don't know how to use it. So we start with the making of a tea. Teas are made from leaves. The second preparation is called a decoction. Decoctions are made from barks and roots. Teas are steeped. Decoctions are simmered. The difference is that the constituents are easy to pull out of leaves but harder to pull out of bark or roots.

Burdock is a perfect herb to taste and then watch a decoction being made from it. After the classes are over, I take the decoction of Burdock to my refrigerator and know that I have just created a vegetarian soup base for my family for the next meal. I can now add anything that I want to this wonderful broth.

The Global.herb V2.0 program found almost 70 different constituents in Burdock. That surely would give a body lots to choose from to create a healthy environment. This same program had a list of things that Burdock was able to help; gout, Sores, boils, Cancer, rheumatism, Skin Disease, arthritis, Catharrh, Eczema, Fever, Colds, Hemorrhoids, Leprosy, Measles, psoriasis, sciatica, tumor, Abscess, Bruises, Cough, Hair-tonic, Lymphatic congestion, Rashes, Snakebite, Swelling, Syphilis, Tonsillitis, Acne, Allergies, Asthma, Blood poison, Burns, Bursitis, Chicken Pox – Blood Cleanser, Chicken Pox-topical for itch, Constipation, Corns, dandruff, Dogbite, Edema, flu, Gonorrhea, Hair loss, Herpes, Hoarseness, Hyperglycemia, Hypoglycemia, Impetigo, Infection, inflammation, Itching, kidney disease, liver problems, Lungs, Parotitis, Pertussis, piles, Pneumonia, Poison Ivy, Poison Oak, Prurigo, Scarlet Fever, Scrofula, Sexual tonic, Skin Diseases, Skin Eruptions, Smallpox, stomachache, sty, Toxic Blood, Tumor – gland, Tumor - Spleen, and Water retention.

That seems like a lot of things to have this wonderful weed work on but in addition the seeds are used for some things and the leaves are used also.

For people who don't want this weed growing in their yard, I suggest that it be used. The root tends to grow up to 16 or more feet long so if you are lucky you might be able to dig the first foot of it and take it out before the second year's growth. The rest of this root will rot and create some very nice soil for the yard.

Another thing to be reminded of is that in the first year this plant looks very much like rhubarb. I always tell my students that when one is harvesting this plant at the end of the first year to make sure that a second year plant is nearby. Burs only grow on second year plants. One might find the skeleton of a burdock plant that died a few years ago in the area with the new plants. Some of these have burs still on them. As much as people dislike this plant, it has been put in our environment for our health.

Calendula

Calendula officinalis

After the seed catalogues have been in our hands for months and we still haven't decided what to put in that little corner of the garden that needs a spot of bright color, let me suggest a marigold called Calendula.

Calendula stands out from the hybrid marigolds in that the flowers have a sunflower look. Other marigolds have many petals all over the composite head of the flower but Calendula has petals only on the fringe or outside of the flower head.

Here is an herb that can cheer us with its pretty orange flowers and do some healing at the same time. Add to that the fact that it can be used in salads and soups, as a pot-herb or just a lovely garnish. We are talking about the multi-pedaled orange-flowered marigolds that were also "used to color cheese" according to Mrs. Grieves, author of A MODERN HERBAL. The yellow color is extracted from the flowers by simmering them.

The flowers and leaves are used for culinary purposes in rice and fish dishes as a garnish. More than that, the flowers were put into broths. Grieves said, "No broths are well made without dried Marigold," and this was without exception in time of plague or pestilence.

Herbalist always refer to this marigold by it botanical name Calendula. These lovelies open to the sun around 9 in the morning and close up again in the afternoon. They can grow up to 28 inches tall with paddle-shaped leaves. The thing that I personally like about them is their hardiness. It seems that they thrive with so little care.

Culpeper mentioned, "The leaves, when chewed, at first communicate a viscid sweetness followed by a strong penetrating taste of a saline nature." It seems the juice containing this pungent matter helps the liver clean toxins out of the body. Plants are so helpful that way.

Culpeper mentioned that by adding vinegar to the leaf matter one could give instant relief to "Hot swelling when bathed with it."

Lesley Bremness, author of the EYEWITNESS HANDBOOK – HERBS, mentions that "research into the ray florets show depilatory effects, potentially useful in face creams." The oils extracted from the macerated flower are very expensive but great for skin problems. One book that I read mentioned that the petals yield a soothing eyewash. This might be because of its antiseptic and antifungal properties.

So far we have only mentioned it being great for the outside of the body but it is great for things like inflamed lymph glands and to stimulate the liver. I have read where one can use it to soothe stomach pains.

I checked Dr. James A. Duke's Database on Calendula and found so many properties in this plant, but mainly in its flowers that are: Antitumor or Anticancer. He uses words like Cancer Preventive, Cardioprotective, Antiviral, Candidicide along with fungicide. There are many properties in this little sunny flower that one could use to stay healthy.

David Christopher, Director of The School Of Natural Healing, has mentioned that if you are using Echinacea to boost the immune system for some problem, you should only take it for 7 days and then switch to something else like Calendula for the next week.

Many books told about all the things that Calendula could do so I decided to find out what my herbal computer program has to say about this. The Globalherb program listed the following things that Calendula is good for: fevers, bruises, toothache, Amenorrhea, Cancer, flu, mouthwash, sprains, bleeding, burns, corns, cuts, earache, hemorrhage, hemorrhoids, jaundice, Lungs, Measles, menses, piles, pyorrhea, Scrofula, skin, Stomachache, Syphilis,

Tuberculosis, ulcerations and warts. All of this from a package of seeds, a first aid kit in itself.

So how do we collect these lovely flowers? One of the nice things is that you are not stripping the whole plant when you harvest just the flowers. When they put new flowers out, we collect them in the morning just after the dew has dried. Then we dry then quickly in an area where they are not touching each other. I like to lay them on a lined cookie sheet and turn the oven on warm. I put a wooden spoon in the door so the moisture can escape. Another way is to put them in a food drier. I store them in a colored glass jar until I am ready to use them.

Maybe it is time to order your seeds and enjoy the "Sunshine" of the Marigold?

Cascara Sagrada
Buckthorn (California)

Buckthorns in general are known for being laxatives. Some of them are harder on the body than others so this is why I want to talk about the one that grows all over the Western United States. It can be found from Idaho to the Pacific and down into California and Mexico.

Before I do this, I would like to remind the reader that Buckthorns grow everywhere, just not the Cascara Sagrada variety. In the state that I live in, there is a war against Buckthorns. It seems that it is an alien plant to this area and the purists want only native plants. My feeling on this is that most people living here are not native to this area; they are imports from Europe but have invaded this territory. Yes, my ancestors made changes to the landscape and so does Buckthorn. It will happen, be open to change as life is not static.

With Cascara Sagrada, it is the bark that is used from this plant. It is harvested in the spring and summer and dried for three of more years. As it ages, it becomes milder.

I would never purchase an herbal laxative that didn't contain Cascara because it doesn't act with the plunger-like actions that other laxatives have. It works mainly on the large intestines.

It activates the peristaltic muscles to keep things moving. These muscles are the ring-like muscles that encircle the intestines and give it a snake-like action, helping food and waste matter to move forward and out. Because of this action, it is not fast acting and will not cause the person to be housebound. One can stay active and still keep the system working.

Most people feel that if they have one bowel movement a day, then they are "regular". This just isn't true. We have three meals a day and snacks but only one evacuation? Something is very wrong.

When there is a new baby with a fully functioning body, every time that it is fed, it needs to have a diaper change.

So too when people eat three meals a day, there should be two or more evacuations per day to keep that person healthy.

When bolus (Clumps) of food matter sit in the intestines for a long period of time, the cells boarding this start to get unhealthy. We see the beginning of Crohn's disease, colitis, and Cancers.

The decaying food will create a very gassy situation that cannot be handled by the release of some of this gas. It tends to migrate to the body cavity and creates much pain. The organs will try to absorb and release some of this to help get it out of the body but the amount of work created by not having a functioning body is putting a strain on all the systems.

When I am very busy and find myself not functioning the way I should, I take a capsule containing Cascara Sagrada bark as its "active ingredient" and know that my body will respond. I can take this before I go to bed knowing that I won't have to get up in the middle of the night. I can take it before I get in the car, knowing that I won't have to rush to find a facility. It really does do the job and works *with* my body.

Catnip

Nepeta cataria

Catnip or Catmint, as it is called, has been used worldwide for thousands of years as a medicinal herb. It was an emigrant from Europe where it was used as a beverage. In Old England it was the beverage of choice until the trade routes made green tea and black tea more prevalent. David Christopher, director of the School of Natural Healing, tells about a Mrs. Bardwell who writes in her book THE HERB GARDEN, "Catnip tea was more wholesome to the British Empire than the Black tea with all the sugar that they needed to make it palatable. Catnip has a mildly sweet flavor all by itself."

On page 260 of his book, THE SCHOOL OF NATURAL HEALING, Dr. John Christopher lists the therapeutic actions of Catnip as: "Aromatic, Relaxant, Diffusive, Stimulant, Diaphoretic, Emmenagogue (herbs that are female correctives to the reproductive organs), Antispasmodic, Nervine (herbs that are tonic and healing to the nerves), Sedative, Carminative (herbs containing a volatile oil that excites intestinal peristalsis and relieves and promotes the expulsion of gas), Anodyne (herbs that relieve pain), Refrigerant, antacid." From all of that you can imagine that this little plant can handle a lot of problems. How do plants do this? They do this because they don't contain one compound like a drug would to handle just one thing; they are composed of a balance of nutriments. No, the active ingredient might not be in the amount that the pharmacist would prefer, but in its own subtle way it gets the job done. It might not do what it is supposed to do in 10 minutes but it will work without the side effects of inorganic chemicals.

This plant is so mild that it has been used by mothers of children for a very long time. By making a tea of Catnip and giving it to a baby even though it is only days or weeks old, it will relieve Colic. It can be given with a teaspoon to do its work. Mom and Dad can go back to sleep and so will baby. Dr. Christopher, found that by adding a little fennel, this tea worked even better for adults at dispelling gas.

Another use for Catnip tea is to rub some on the gums of babies when they are teething.

As much as it has a relaxing effect on people, it seems to have the opposite effect on cats. It is almost like a "fix" for cats but research has shown that only 2/3 of all cats are affected. This includes all of the cat family from house cats to tigers and lions. I dried some catnip in a plant press and found the press torn apart and the catnip broken into pieces by my cats. I guess mine are in that 2/3 percent.

According to David, the American Medical Association in JAMA 1969 (Their major publication) claimed that Catnip produced Marijuana-like effects. The wire service picked up this story and according to David, pet stores had a run on cat toys. Contrary to this claim, Catnip is not hallucinogenic.

Catnip was registered from 1842 to 1882 in the US Pharmacopia, thus registering it as a medicinal herb, as it should be. According the Daniel Mowrey in THE SCIENTIFIC VALIDATION OF HERBAL MEDICINE, it has been found to have Antibiotic properties.

This is why it is so useful for colds and flu, but according to the Globalherb V2.0 computer program it can even be used to prevent Chicken Pox. This was a little strong for me but their reference for this came from Steven Horne's NATURE'S FIELD book published in 1991. David Christopher has suggested mixing it with Saffron to handle Smallpox and Scarlet Fever. Looks like Catnip is more powerful than we give it credit.

Another thing that Catnip tea is good for is to cut phlegm in the bronchial system. Native Americans smoked Catnip for asthma and bronchial problems. In Europe they would mix it with honey to create a cough medicine.

Catnip can be used to expel worms from the intestine by making an enema of the tea. Dr. John Christopher called this an injection.

Herbalists do not puncture their skin with needles. Once you break the hematic seal, your body is exposed to substances that are not in its best interest. (It is the job of the skin to seal the blood from foreign matter.) The premise is that the vaccines will get the immune system to "kick" in and try to get rid of the invaders. The bad part is that foreign proteins along with other things are introduced beyond the skin barrier and into the blood system. (For interesting reading on what is in vaccines read Dr. Leonard G. Horowitz's book called EMERGING VIRUSES, AIDs & EBOLA- NATURE, ACCIDENT OR INTENTIONAL?)

The foreign substances that are introduced into the blood system are not all killed. Some are parked or find their way to a specific organ and we have the beginnings of autoimmune diseases.

One of the cautions that I ran into regarding Catnip was that is shouldn't be taken during pregnancy as it promotes menses. According to David Christopher that is what all the books say but his wife, Fawn said that because it is a relaxant, when she was pregnant and started spotting, she made a cup of Catnip Tea and sat back to relax. The Antispasmodic effects "Will calm the uterus and stop cramping during menstruation," according to the Christophers.

Along with all that we have mentioned about this little wild mint, (and it grows everywhere) it will also aid digestion. Many years ago a friend of mine from England told me that the way the British stay slim is to follow a meal with a nice mint tea. I guess that is because Catnip relaxes the body along with assisting with the meal. I have an idea that Catnip is now on the dinner mint list.

Cayenne

Capsicum Frutescens

The pepper family is a wonderful herbal family that takes in all the members from Sweet Green Peppers to hot Cayenne Peppers. Some of the hot peppers have the ability to burn the skin but for the most part, what you purchase in the store will not be that hot and will give the body a lot of benefits. Dr. John R. Christopher once mentioned that a person could stand all day on a clove of garlic in bare feet and nothing would happen but if they stood on a hot Cayenne, they would find the skin affected.

Let's start with its ability to balance out blood pressure. In our family we use Cayenne capsules like other families use aspirin, to handle headaches. A lot of headaches are due to increased blood pressure and Cayenne will not allow the pressure to be more in one place (the head) than in any other place in the body. Headaches come from a lot of different things so we are just talking about blood pressure at this time.

My husband called from work and it seemed that his secretary had a headache. All he had was Cayenne in his desk drawer. He wanted to know if he could give her one, she has ulcers. I mentioned that he could and that the Cayenne might kill Helicobacter pylori (H. Pylori), the bacteria that causes ulcers, in any case it might cauterize the wound. I did tell him to remind her that it would create some real discomfort in her stomach; most people don't want help that hurts.

Side story is that the H. Pylori doesn't like an alkaline environment but does like acid. The mouth with its saliva is an alkaline environment and would have killed this bacteria had it spent more time there than in the acid of the stomach. This person is not taking time to eat properly and chewing foods into small particles while mixing the saliva with it, thus allowing this acid-loving bacteria through to the stomach. Bacteria have a very narrow comfort zone and if we can kill the acid-loving ones in the mouth and the alkaline-loving ones in the stomach, we will find that our bodies don't have to work hard at all to keep us healthy.

Dr. Christopher mentioned that the ability to balance of blood pressure would be helpful for someone that had been injured and was bleeding. By giving that person a Cayenne capsule or infusion of Cayenne, the blood pressure would balance out and there would be more time to get that person medical help with less bleeding. He also mentioned that if one were having a heart attack, by using Cayenne and balancing the pressure out, the damage would be minimalized before getting medical assistance. My family has a history of heart problems so I carry Cayenne capsules with me all the time.

While attending classes in Utah, one of the things that students were asked to participate in was the Cayenne test. Powdered Cayenne was put into the palm of our hand, and then we were told to cover one nostril with the other hand and snort the powder. This gets the Cayenne powder to the sinuses and starts the healing. Most of us have more mucus than is needed in the sinuses area. Cayenne cuts this and starts the healing process by bring blood to these cells. Yes, it is best to do this with a box of tissue because one's nose and eyes will run for a very long time and you will feel the mucus draining down the throat.

After doing this for a while, Cayenne is something that one gets used to and there are side benefits from this. The optic nerve is very close to the sinus area. I found that I didn't need my glasses after I cleaned the toxins from the sinus area.

In his book ALKALIZE OR DIE, Dr. Baroody Says, "Cayenne Pepper – A miracle food! Cayenne *heals* the body. Black pepper, an acid-former, irritates the stomach, while cayenne is especially good for stomach ulcers. It can be eaten in pods, as a powdered condiment, or taken as a nutritional supplement to stimulate the entire endocrine system. Take 1 to 2 capsules, 3 times a day. " On the Alkaline scale, it rates as a 7.0; this is very, very alkaline.

Perhaps this is why it is good for a heart patient because when one goes to the hospital, they give an alkaline solution to the heart patients for the same reason that we suggested.

Cayenne is loaded with vitamins and minerals. I found over 200 different chemicals in this one herb. With all of them working simultaneously, is it any wonder that this herb is so powerful.

Cayenne has been used for Stomach problems, Gas, Gastrointestinal tract aches and cramps. It has been used as a gargle for sore throats and as a counterirritant for rheumatic arthritic pain.

Because this herb has some powerful effects on the system, I feel it is ideal to talk about how to take herbs. A lot of people tell me that they can't "take" herbs and when I ask them why, they tell me that the herb "backs up" on them and they taste it all day. This is because no one has taught them how to take an herb. We are so used to popping a pill with a sip of water and expecting it to go to work for us. Herbs don't work that way. Let's say we just took a capsule of any herb with a sip of water. This capsule goes to our stomach and sits on top of the acid that is naturally there. The water that we sipped this with has filtered through the system. This capsule finally opens, leaving all of its contents just sitting there on top of the stomach acid. A little at a time this will assimilate into the acid but to properly take an herb, one needs to make a tea out of it.

To do this with a capsule is to take the herbal capsule with the sip of water, wait for a short time and then drink the rest of the glass of water. Now the herb will be made into a usable tea and will readily enter the rest of the body to go to work for us.

The major problem with herbal health is that we have never been taught about it in any of our education. We aren't even told about its benefits as foods, let alone the healing benefits.

At an organic farm, I was attending one of their public functions, one of the interns working there knew that I was an herbalist and came running into the barn where I was talking to some of the other visitors. He told me that I should come as there was an emergency. I went with him to the man that had just swallowed a hornet from his soda can. It had stung his esophagus. I took them to the garden and pulled up some Plantain and Chickweed as both of these will pull toxins out of the skin. I told him to chew on these but only swallow the juice, not the plants. Then I had him spit the plants out and gave him a sip of Cayenne water that I had made from a capsule that I had with me. He told me that it burned all the way down. I nodded knowing that it was pulling blood to that area to help from inside of the body also. I told him that if at any time he was having a problem swallowing or breathing, he should head to the nearest emergency room.

I kept watching him and his family as they continued to go on the hayrides and play the games. They stuck around for a long time. Weeks later I asked the owner of the farm if she had ever heard from that man about what had happened. She told me that she hadn't. So I asked if she would mind if I called him and did she have his address. She gave me a phone number and I called. I told the man who I was and asked how he was doing. He told me that he was very angry with me because the rest of that whole day his throat and chest burned from that Cayenne.

What can I say? Some people don't know how close to having a real problem that they have just avoided. I didn't mention anything to him other than I was concerned.

Whether or not we like what and how they work for us, Herbs do work! They want to do what they can to help. Cayenne can do so much that it should be in every household.

> I cannot teach anyone anything.
> I can only make them think.
> Socrates

Chamomile

Anthemis nobilis

I got a call one day from a lady whose three-year old was covered with hives. This poor little dear had them everywhere. She was so uncomfortable. One of the first things that I did was confirm that it was hives. The Mother told me that they had been to the doctor, he told her it was hives and had given her some salve but it wasn't working.

I went into Dr. James A. Duke's book, THE GREEN PHARMACY to see what he used on hives and he suggested Chamomile as it contains at least seven (7) Antihistaminic chemicals.

So this little girl was given Chamomile tincture with a Chamomile tea to wash it down. Her mother told me that at first it got worse but within hours she could see the results. A lot of people call this a 'healing crisis'; that's when things get worse before they get better. It is usually at this point that people decide that herbs don't work for them. By the next day this little girl has just a few spots on her and wanted to go to her swimming lessons.

According to what I read, Chamomile is great at stimulating the liver to throw toxins out. Here is one really safe herb. We use it mostly for stomach or intestinal complaints but it is also used in skin creams and lotions for its Antibacterial properties.

I checked into some of the things that Chamomile is capable of doing and found that it is loaded with Antibacterial and Antiinflammatory properties. It also has a fair number of constituents that are Antiviral, even found one that was Antirhinovirol. (This is the cold and flu virus that is advertised all the time.)

37

Chamomile is a fun thing to grow in one's garden. It has these wonderful small white flowers. The best part is that you are using the flowers to make your medicine. So many plants give everything for our healing to the point of having to dig them up and use their roots but not so with Chamomile. It can continue to grow and put out more flowers.

We can use these flowers to make tinctures within 14 days. Or we can use the flower as a tea by pouring hot water over them and allowing them to steep for 5 to 10 min. (I use distilled water so that the constituents can be pulled into the water faster without having to deal with all of the calcium and iron that is in my tap water.) Another thing that can be made from these flowers, are skin salves or body lotions.

When people read about herbs the first thing that they want to know is, "So how can I use this?" I want to say, any way you want to. Herbs are foods so ingest them or use some of the methods that I have just pointed out.

This last summer, I had to take many small Chamomile plants out of the bed that they are growing in. It was taking over and not respecting the space of the plants around them. Once you get it started and don't harvest every flower, you are going to have more next year. Nature gives us abundance.

According to NUTRITIONAL HERBOLOGY written by Mark Pedersen, the flowers actually contain the following: aluminum, ash, calcium, chromium, cobalt, iron, magnesium, manganese, niacin, phosphorus, potassium, protein, riboflavin, selenium, silicon, sodium, thiamine, tin, Vitamin A, Vitamin C and zinc. He mentions that it is very high in niacin, a substance that tends to care for the nervous system, making this a very sedative herb or Antispasmodic herb.

I want to discuss the first thing on this list. We have been told over and over again that aluminum is something that creates brain problems...Alzheimer's? This needs to be corrected! Aluminum is needed to make the connections in the brain but only if it is organic aluminum. How can this be? It is because organic chemicals have the ability to cross the blood/brain barrier both ways. Inorganic chemicals do not have this ability. They are stuck once they get in there and if a lot of in-organics are going in and not coming out, we have a problem. The brain knows that it needs aluminum and because we are not eating foods with organic aluminum in them, the body will steal the aluminum from our soda cans or the foil that we put on our foods, all waste products of the mining industry. When we give it organic aluminum, it doesn't steal and can recognize the difference.

My computer program, Globalherb V2.0 tells me that Chamomile is good for; colic, colds, earache, indigestion, spasms, jaundice, swelling, toothache, bruises, fever, prevention of gangrene, gas, inflammation, Insomnia, Neuralgia, bronchitis, corns, cramps, gastritis, nervousness, sores, leg ulcers, abscess, alcoholism, allergies, Anxiety, lack of appetite, Cancer, liver cancer, poor circulation, colitis, constipation, Crohn's disease, diarrhea, and gastric ulcers.

If you have never had a cup of Chamomile Tea, you must be sitting back right now wondering just how this mild tea is going to start working on any or all of this. It will because all of the things available in this plant are designed for your health. They allow your body to receive the nutrition that isn't in your daily meals or the snacks that you allow yourself.

Let me suggest that you make a cup of Chamomile tea right now and relax while allowing your body to go to work for you. I think you will have a very pleasant day if you do.

Chickweed

Stellaria media

I have read that there isn't any part in the world where Chickweed doesn't grow. Mrs. Grieves, a noted herbalist talked about it being native to all temperate regions, even into arctic regions. It is one of the most common weeds and one that we pull out of our gardens regularly.

After reading about where it grows, one would think that this is a very hardy plant when in fact it is tiny and frail looking. Chickweed has leaves that are succulent and egg-shaped, about one inch long and one-half inch wide with a little point on the end of each leaf. The plant is usually pale green and smooth. The flowers are located by some of the upper leaves and these little white flowers look like tiny white stars.

Traditional Chickweed has been used for inflammations, boils, cough, eyes, hemorrhoids, hoarseness, rheumatism, skin disease, blood toxicity, bronchitis, colds, constipation, pleurisy, sores, tumors, burns, Cancer, Crohn's disease, deafness, fever, wounds, abscesses, acne, allergies, asthma, bronchial congestion, cellulite, cholesterol, colitis, Eczema, fracture, gout, hay fever, infection, itchy skin, mucus, obesity, plague, psoriasis, rabies, spasms, and Stomach ulcers. All of this information was found in the Globalherb computer program by Blake.

I haven't tried it for all of these conditions but I will tell you some of the ways that I have used Chickweed.

My eleven year old cousin, James had large welts all over him where he had been bitten by mosquitoes while we were bike riding.

When we got home, I put two handfuls of Chickweed into the bathtub and turned on the water. I told him not to pull the plug when he got out but to soak in this Chickweed tea. When I saw him next, the welts were gone and just the quarter-sized red circles were still all over him. The redness left within a few hours. He told me that when he stepped in, the itching stopped immediately. Chickweed had pulled out the toxin and allowed his body to heal.

My Father-in-law was bothered by Shingles. If you have ever had them you know that they itch like mad. I told him that when I had Shingles, I used Chickweed tea. I had my husband bring in a handful of Chickweed that I then put into a kettle of water. I simmered this for a while and allowed it to cool. Using a cloth, I bathed the area that was bothering me and the itching stopped as the tea touched it. My Father-in-law was so happy to hear this. Chickweed only handles the symptoms of Shingles; there are other things that get it out of the body so that it can't reoccur.

I have two ragdoll cats. The younger cat has matte eyes all the time. We think she has a chronic sinus infection. The Vet tells me that cats with long hair tend to have matte eyes so we wash her eyes out from time to time with Chickweed tea. She doesn't like it but will put up with us. I decided to see if this tea stings or what she might not like about it so I washed my eyes out with it. (I love to be a guinea pig on things like this.) I found out that it is so mild to the eyes; one could wash a sty on a baby if necessary. Because of its ability to pull fat and toxins out, it is perfect to use for sties.

So it was just getting her eyes washed that she didn't like. One could use this as a wash for any facial swellings or redness.

There are many salves that are made with Chickweed in them for its Antiitching property along with being Antibacterial and soothing to the skin.

Chickweed is found in a lot of herbal loss weight products for this very reason. It attaches to fat in the intestinal tract and brings it along with it out of the body. It can make the stomach feel full and not allow one to over eat. As part of a salad, it has very little taste so can be combined with just about anything and with any dressing.

The Globalherb program also gave me a breakdown on some of the constituents in this little plant.   I was impressed with the almost 50 things that they mentioned; Everything from Vitamin C (and the printout states "lots" behind this one as it does behind Vitamin A and B), to niacin, calcium (lots), iron (lots), manganese and magnesium, phosphorus, potassium, protein, and zinc. I can see that a salad made out of this weed sure would give the body a lot of choices to build with.

The next time you are weeding in your garden and you come across this wonderful plant, make sure that you set it aside to be taken into the house to be washed and ready for your next meal, salad or even in a sandwich. You will be doing yourself a big favor.

ComFrey
Symphytum officinale

On one of my first visits to Boulder Colorado, attending Hanna Kroeger's seminar, I was introduced to a plant that I had never heard of before. That wasn't strange, as there are some 200,000 medicinal plants and I was just starting to learn about them at that time. The best part was that after the seminar, Hanna's son went to the garden and dug up a Comfrey plant for me to take home. I was honored.

I brought this plant home and put it in my back yard. It has large hairy, pointed leaves with beautiful blue bell-like flowers on the top. It grows about 2 to almost 3 feet high in my yard.

Since I planted it, I have learned a lot about it. One thing is that once it is planted, it wants to grow there forever. I have moved it twice. In both instances I have had to talk to the plant to get it to let go of its former place. The last move was to move it deeper into the hedge so that when it gets really tall; its leaves aren't over the grass area so that it gets mowed all the time.

During the lecture in Colorado, Hanna mentioned that Comfrey was wonderful for rebuilding cells. She didn't specify which cells at that time but I have come to take that as all cells. Because it rebuilds cells quickly, it has gotten the nick-name of "People Putty." What an appropriate name. Perhaps that is why the other common names for this plant are Knitbone, Bruisewort, and Knitback.

Dr. John R. Christopher quoted a lot from one of his mentors, Dr. Shook. According to what I read Dr. Shook said, "It does not seem to matter much which part of the body is broken, either

43

internally or externally; comfrey will heal it quickly. It is a great cell proliferant and new cell grower, it grows new flesh and bone alike, stops hemorrhage, and is wonderful for coughs, soothing and healing inflamed tissues in a most remarkable manner."

Another thing that was mentioned by Dr. Christopher is the respiratory system. The lungs are able to heal well using this plant. It acts as an expectorant with soothing effects it reduces irritation.

Everyone that I researched this plant with reminded me that the root and young leaves contain a toxic alkaloid, which is said to create liver damage *if taken in large amounts*. But in the same articles it is mentioned that the root and the young leaves would be good for ulcerous wounds.

Most people that work with Comfrey tend to put it in combinations. Combinations are made by finding herbs that would be most helpful for the area involved, a transporter (something that has an affinity for the specific area.) and then the herbs that would supply that area with the most nutriments for healing.

It has been stated that certain plants tend to gravitate to specific areas of the body. I have been told that they think they can get out that way. As an example, Parsley tends to go for the kidneys while Rosemary might head for the brain. Why they do this is unknown.

Comfrey has a demulcent mucilage presents which is helpful with things like hiatus hernia and ulcerative colitis.

Christopher Products has created a blend of herbs that was called Bone, Flesh and Cartilage (BF&C). I liked that name but it has since been changed to Complete Tissue. It has been made into an ointment and its uses are endless.

I used this ointment on a young boy who fell out of a tree and tore his face. With the help of comfrey that will repair and "guard against scar tissue developing incorrectly", according to David Hoffmann in his book AN ELDERS' HERBAL; it did just what he said it would do. This child has little or no scaring.

A nurse, who broke her arm, was able to heal it in four weeks instead of the usual six weeks by applying the ointment topically and ingesting this formula in capsule form. Thus she healed from both the inside and the outside of her body.

When sores get to the scab stage, it is time to switch to the Complete Tissue formula to complete the healing. The nutrition will pass through the scab and speed up the healing process.

So far we have only talked about what Comfrey can do for human bodies but I did say that it was a cell proliferant and I meant it. I dry some of the leaves and when I am repotting my house plants, I mix these leaves into the soil to give my plants a real boost of energy.

Next, I wanted to check in with Dr. James Duke and his wonderful database to see what things this herb is capable of doing. The amazing thing is that in the leaf area, Dr. Duke didn't have a whole lot to tell me but when it came to the root of Comfrey, what isn't it able to do? The list went from Antiaging to Antiviral and everything in between. I have always talked about how plants achieve a balance, and I even found two components in these roots that were Antiproliferant.

After looking at Duke's list, I went to my Globalherb program to see what they had to say about Comfrey. Their list was just as impressive with: bruises, cough, diarrhea, anemia, fractures, hemorrhage, inflammation, sores, ulcers, boils, bronchitis, Cancer, dysentery, leucorrhea, rupture, swelling, acne, arthritis, asthma, burns, catarrh, Diabetes, gangrene, gout, hay fever, sore breasts, sprains and another page and a half of things that it would be happy to work on.

One must remember that unlike what most of us think, that more is better; when it comes to herbs a little goes a long way. This is a very safe herb if used correctly and that means not to overdo it.

All herbs have something to give us if we use common sense. We have not been trained to think like this. If we have a headache, we think that if one aspirin is good then two should be twice as good. It is the same way that we think about herbal tea. We like our coffee strong so it will really be good, so how can a weak, see-through tea be helpful?

When making a tea out of an herb it is best to make it with distilled water. Distilled water is hungry water and for all practical purposes does not have all the minerals that our tap water has. Because it has room for all the constituents contained in the herb, it is ready to pull these into the water that you will be ingesting.

It is for the reason that has just been pointed out that I don't like to see people doing the same things all the time. One wouldn't eat peanut butter for every meal so why would one take a comfrey tea or capsule all the time. By doing different herbs, we give the body different constituents to choose from. This is how healing really takes place.

Herbs don't heal, they give the body the building blocks to rebuild and Comfrey is a great rebuilder.

Dandelion

Taraxacum officinale

Did you know that there is a war going on in your neighborhood, and it is chemical warfare? Most of us haven't a clue what is happening right under our noses. Who is benefiting from this war, Mr. and Mrs. Perfect? Who is it hurting, almost everyone and everything thing in the neighborhood. Do you know people who are allergic to a lot of things? Maybe you know someone who has asthma? A lot of my friends have taken the carpeting out of their houses in favor of hardwood floors because of all the allergies but don't think twice about what they are doing to their lawns.

In this chapter I want to talk about Dandelions. Most people have someone come in and spray to get rid of them. These companies do this at a rate of four or more times a summer to keep Dandelions from messing up their perfect yard. If they would only realize that Dandelions are helping the yard to stay healthy. These colorful plants are loaded with the ability to help everything around them, us included.

History teaches us that the new and smaller leaves can be used in salads. These salads are loaded with Vitamins A and C along with minerals such as organic chromium, organic calcium, organic potassium and organic selenium. You will even find organic zinc in trace amounts. The leaves are a powerful diuretic and are used to treat urinary disorders without depleting the body of potassium. These same leaves detoxify the blood and are therefore used for acne and eczema.

The leaves have trace amounts of all sorts of good things. The body does not need a whole capsule of selenium or most of the other things that we get at the health food store, these leaves are perfect. We need traces to stay healthy just like these plants. If they get too much of something, they are out of balance just like we get when we do too much of anything.

Jethro Kloss, an herbalist that grew up in Wisconsin, mentioned that Dandelion "has a beneficial effect on female organs along with increasing the activity of the liver, pancreas and spleen." It is especially great when dealing with an enlargement of the liver or spleen.

The roots nourish and cleanse the kidneys, skin and even affect the heart, due to its blood purifying properties. Historically the root has been used to reduce inflammation, correct conditions in rheumatic joints and through the liver, clean up jaundice and gall stones.

At our house we use dried Dandelion roots like black pepper on our food. According to one of my mentors, when you use the real Black Pepper, be sure to use it after cooking as the heat changes its chemical properties.

When my mother had a stroke, she "balled" her hand into her shoulder. While doing some research, I found that Rosemary sprigs were placed in Dandelion Wine and made into a tonic to help Queen Victoria's Cousin who had a stroke. We did this and Mom relaxed her hand into her lap. (Rosemary heads for the brain.)

I make Dandelion wine out of the Dandelion petals. Spring is the best time to do this with the abundance of flowers, as one needs a gallon of flower petals. I made it once with the calyx (the green part on the back of the flower) and got a green wine so after that I pulled petals off the flowers. The next step is to pour a gallon of hot water over these petals and let them stand for 12 hours, drain them, saving the liquid and add to only the liquid, 3 pounds of sugar, the juice of one orange and two lemons and a package of yeast. (I use wine yeast for this and the packet tells me that it makes 5 gallons but I only make one so I seal the remaining yeast and refrigerate it for another time.) Now it is time to allow it to ferment.

I don't believe in investing a lot of money in small projects so I use plastic water gallon jugs to process this. I have found a beach balloon at the drug store that has a very large opening, so this is stretched over the mouth of the gallon jug. As my product ferments, the balloon fills with the gas that is being made. When the ball gets about 18 inches in diameter, I put a pin hole in the hard rubber nipple that was designed to tie a rubber band on. When my wine is not able to make enough gas to keep my balloon inflated, it is time to bottle.

At bottling time I taste the wine and decide if it needs help. This last spring I had two jugs going. One came out very dry and the other very sweet so when bottling, these were combined to make the perfect blend. The sterilized bottles and caps have been cooled and are ready to receive the wine.

The last process is to label. I am very big on labeling. I find that many times without labels we forget what we have. When I harvest leaves and dry them, they look nothing like what they did when I picked them and are hard to identify. So I put them into a paper bag and write on the bag that this is Dandelion roots or whatever it is. Labeling is so important.

I need to talk about the paper bag. Most people think that you dry herbs by hanging them upside down in a cool dry place. If I did that, I would be processing all sorts of bugs. I love bugs and they have a place in my world but not in the herbs that I plan to make medicine with. So my herbs get put into large paper bags and then I write what is in there and staple the top together. I shake this bag every so often and turn it to another surface of the bag. Bags have bottoms and four sides. The side that it is laying on will become damp as the moisture is being wicked out of the plant matter. The wet side is now up and will dry allowing more moisture to leave. This way when they are completely dry and I put the plant matter into glass jars for storage, they will not mildew. They have been completely dried.

Back to wine. Wine is great for cooking and drinking and healing. In the cooking process the alcohol is dissipated so even people who can't drink wine, can cook with it and get many benefits from the properties that are left in the foods. My students have sampled my Dandelion wine and I have had no complaints.

The late Hanna Kroeger used Dandelion flowers to clean up Diabetes. In the Globalherb computer program, there is reference given from a book by John Heinerman called *"Science of Herbal Medicine"*, for using Dandelions to heal the pancreas.

Dandelions can do so much more. They have been used to handle age spots, anemia, as an appetite stimulant, arthritis, asthma, blisters, blood cleanser, high blood pressure, gall bladder problems, hepatitis, Hypoglycemia, kidney infections, skin problems and weight loss.

In many countries Dandelions are cultivated as a food. The roots are cooked as a vegetable.

For those who dislike the looks of Dandelion, perhaps taking a page out of David Christopher's book (the director of the School of Natural Healing) and eat the flowers early in the morning before the animals have been around, would keep them from putting their seeds out and making more. If you try them you might understand why bees like them.

No matter how you use Dandelions, they are a harbinger of health. Usually they tell me that there are few if any toxins in the area where they are found. Even Dogs like our yard because we are not at war with the Dandelion.

Echinacea

Echinacea angustifolia

Yesterday was the day to harvest pears. Our pear tree was overloaded and the pears looked wonderful. I had taken some in last week and after allowing them to sit out on the cupboard for about 4 or 5 days, they became soft and yellow and delicious!

In the process of going up the ladder to cut some of the fruit off the tree, I must have taken on a passenger. When I came done to the ground I felt something stinging me so I crushed my pant leg and rushed into the house to see what bit me. When I got inside, I found a very large red spot with a raised area that covered a two inch round section of my leg. I dragged out my Echinacea tincture and put some of a dropperful on my leg while rubbing it in to keep it in that area. I did this a second and third time and then I went back out to finish my work. By the time I was done and came in, the area was not raised but still red. That was yesterday; today it is just pink and itches a bit.

Echinacea is a native to my area and it has been used a lot. Most people think of it being used only to boost the immune system but it has many uses.

While we are talking about bites, I must mention spider bites because they are very different from other insect bites. Spiders inject an enzyme that breaks down the cell walls and this is why when one is bitten by a spider, the red streak starts up or down that body part. Echinacea when dropped on the bite of a spider will stop the enzymatic action and contain the problem.

Echinacea will put the immune system on high alert but will only do this for about a week. After a week one must switch to another herb for this same action. A couple that might be used for this purpose are Chinese Astragalus or Calendula flowers.

The American Indians would chew on the root of Echinacea for relief from respiratory afflictions.

In Germany there are many salves, tinctures and extracts made using Echinacea. The claim has been made that it is Antiviral and can be used for virus infections as well as for bacteria. Most Doctors only have Antibiotics although they are starting to get Antiviral products on the market.

I just researched Dr. James Duke's Database to see what else this wonderful herb can do. I found that the plant contains about 120 different constituents and that the root (I make my tincture from the root) contains 70 of those constituents. A lot of these constituents would be things that you recognize such as chromium, iron, manganese, niacin, selenium, zinc and many more. All of these are organic so that our organic bodies can use them as needed. That is a lot of things to put in balance and if they aren't in balance with each other, the plant will die.

Now what are these constituents capable of doing for me? Using only the ones in my tincture, they are capable of so many things that I will just mention the things that more than two of these constituents are capable of doing. They are: Antiallergenic, Antiacne, Antiaging, Antialzheimeran, Antiarthritic, Antiasthmatic, Antibacterial, Anticataract, Antidementia, Antidiabetic, Antidote for aluminum and lead, Antiinflammatory, Antileukemic, Antimigraine, Antioxidant, Antiparkinsonian, Antiseptic, Antistaph, Antistress, Antisyndrome X, Antiviral, Cancer preventive, Cardio protective, fungicide, sedative, and Vasodilator.

That is a lot of hard work and it is all in a bottle for me without side effects. This pharmacy is growing in your front yard. No more pills and shots for your family when Dr. Mom gets busy. These remedies can be made in your kitchen.

I did read an article about the toxicity of Echinacea and it mentioned that this herb if given to the power of 50 in an injection could be toxic. This makes me laugh because as an herbalist, I don't believe in shots; I could see if one would give a shot that has 50 times the amount of that herbalist would suggest, could and would be toxic. When these herbs are tested on animals, these animals are given the equivalent of eating 10 meals at one sitting. All of us would have an adverse reaction to something like that.

To make a tincture one needs to have the herb of choice, in this case it is Echinacea Root. In herbal language this is called the marc. (The marc can be any herbal part, be it root or plant.) When using root material, one needs to chop it into small pieces. When using leaves this isn't that necessary.

Now we need some form of alcohol as a preservative. In herbal language this is called the menstrum. (Menstrums come in all forms from water, to oil or even vinegar) I use 100 proof vodka. Why 100 proof? Because it is 50 % water and 50 % alcohol, it doesn't have fillers like 80 proof does. One can use a brand of vegetable alcohol called Everclear. Vodka is a vegetable alcohol too.

Step one is to put the herb into a glass bottle, filling it one fourth to one third full of plant material.

Step two is to pour the alcohol over the plant material, filling the bottle to the top.

Step three is to cap and shake the bottle every day for fourteen days. This makes sure that the plant matter doesn't settle to the bottom of the bottle. The object is for the alcohol to pull out the constituents that will be used for healing from the plant material. (Hence the small pieces of root.)

Step four is to strain the plant material out of the preservative after the 14 days and return the preservative that contains all the helpful constituents to the bottle, putting some of it into a dropper bottle to be used as needed in the medicine chest. Don't forget to label all your bottles.

Dr. John R. Christopher said that we should eat from our own back yard. This means that foods grown at our latitude, our longitude and our altitude have the right vibration for our body cells. Perhaps that is why herb books never mention bananas. Most herb books were written for the people of Europe and North America. I find that most interesting.

Stay healthy and use what is growing in your own back yard to do this.

Fenugreek

Trigonella Foenum

My sister Betty spent the summer with us and we had a great time. Betty has diabetes so she has to keep checking her blood sugar all the time. I am glad that she does this to take care of herself.

Sometime in the middle of the summer, she noticed that her blood sugar was high and she mentioned this to me. I asked what _she_ was going to do about this. She mentioned that she could take a walk and sometimes that brings the blood sugar down but if it didn't then I could give her a shot. Sorry, I don't give shots nor do I take them.

I have been taught that my body is hermetically sealed. This means that I have a barrier between my insides and my outsides. There is skin everywhere to keep me from being exposed to anything. I bleed out, not in so that my blood supply is protected from contaminates. To purposely put something foreign under my skin, breaking this protective barrier would not be in my best interest.

So the first thing that I did for my sister was to put some powdered Cinnamon into a glass of water. They don't like to mix so it takes a while to get the cinnamon wet. I told her to drink this when it is damp and in the meanwhile I would soak some Fenugreek. I went into my files to show her information about Fenugreek and that it has been known to bring the blood sugar down 54% in a little while. Not sure where that figure came from but I think it was in my notes from the School of Natural Healing.

To our surprise (because I never had to use this before) after eating only a teaspoon of the Fenugreek seeds, her blood sugar was down to normal. After that she wouldn't go anywhere without it.

The seeds themselves are very hard when dried but after soaking them for a few hours; they are soft and chewy like Millet. They have a grain flavor similar to oat groats or Wheat berries.

Not a bad flavor at all. Everywhere that I read about fenugreek, they talk about a bitter taste but I have eaten it many times and have tasted bitterness only when it has been sitting around for a long time. My sister did have some soaking for many days so we dumped them and soaked some more.

In one article it did talk about the down side of this herb and that being that if you eat too much, one of the many constituents, Sotolone will perfume both your sweat and urine. They will smell like maple syrup or curry, neither of which sounds like a major problem.

Not knowing a lot about this plant, I headed for Wikipedia to learn more about it. It goes by many names in other countries and is used extensively in Europe and Asia. In these countries they treat digestion problems, sinus, lung congestion and infections with this plant. It is also used to reduce inflammation and promote milk production in lactating women.

In Ethiopia and India, it is a natural Diabetic medicine.

I decided to find out what in it is helpful for Diabetes. Checking only the constituents of the seeds in Dr. James A. Duke's Database, I found that arginine, chromium, fiber, magnesium, manganese, niacin, Quercetin and zinc had Antidiabetic properties. Even that is a lot for tiny seeds.

Being Antidiabetic wasn't the only ability that these tiny seeds are capable of doing. There have been two recent studies (Baschel – 2003 and Srinivas- 2005) showing that this plant has major Anticancer abilities. I found the seeds to be Antioxident, Antibacterial, Antistress, Antiinflammatory, Antiviral and much more…like helping the liver, lowering cholesterol, and triglycerides.

These seeds have been found in many archeological digs and have been carbon dated to 4000 BC. They are linked to prosperity in the Jewish religion and are eaten at Rosh Hashanah to bring good fortune to the New Year.

If you haven't tried Fenugreek, don't do it because it will keep your blood sugar down but use it as a grain in stews and soups. I read once that where we used to eat a great variety of foods every year, we now eat the same few foods over and over. It is good to add something new to your diet, giving the body more choices and combinations to work from. As you know by the list that I mentioned for Diabetes, there is a lot of nutrition that you will be giving your body with this addition to your food supply. There were also 20 to 30 more things in these seeds that did other things than help with blood sugar. Enjoy a new food.

Feverfew

Chrysanthemum parthenium

Yesterday a friend called to tell me that she had a Migraine headache. Never having experienced this, it is hard to imagine but they tell me that it is the granddaddy of all headaches.

With all of that in mind, it was time to write about a Chrysanthemum plant that is in blossom at this time called Feverfew. One of the interesting things that I have read about this plant is that it is commonly consumed by chewing fresh leaves. Another things that I learned was that if one is subjected to Migraines, Feverfew should be taken daily instead of when one feels the Migraine coming on.

I did find a lot of components in Feverfew that were Antimigraine, but there were a lot that were also Vasodilators. I suppose that if you put those two properties together, you can really relieve a lot of problems.

Research has actually shown that it is better at reducing inflammation and fevers than even aspirin.

In Europe it was used for relief of depression, nausea and arthritic pain. It is said to be a general tonic for the body.

One of the other bits of information that I found was that it relieves asthma attacks. I did find some antihistamine properties in this herb also.

In folklore, plants were usually named for what they were most used for and this one got the name of Feverfew as it was used for fevers long before it was used as a headache remedy.

Sometimes it was use to help with delivering the afterbirth in childbirth. It was great for hot swellings (inflammations.)

The GLOBALHERB program has a list of things that Feverfew is good for. They are: fever, colds, colic, hysteria, indigestion, nerve pressure, amenorrhea, anemia, arthritis, Cancer, diarrhea, dizziness, dyspepsia, earache, excess heat, flatulence, flu, Hayfever, headache, insect bites, Migraine, psoriasis, spasms, tension, wheezing, and worms. I would say that is a lot for one small plant to take on.

Culpepper wrote "Troubled with melancholy and heaviness or sadness of spirit?" when he was talking about Feverfew as a remedy for depression.

Dr. Michael Murray, author of THE HEALING POWER OF HERBS, mentioned that, "the 6-month Migraine studies made no report of toxic reactions in patients taking feverfew. Feverfew has been used by large numbers of people for many years without reports of toxicity. Chewing the leaves, however, may result in ulcerations, and some sensitive persons will develop an exudative dermatitis from external contact."

As for growing this plant, it tends to reseed itself and it tried to take over my peppermint bed this year. As a gardener, one must always set limits and this is a plant that needs to be limited.

We are given abundance.

Garlic

Allium sativum

How many people can predict the weather? Probably more than we think. Some people "feel" that a storm is heading our way with their bodies. This is real, they really feel when the pressure drops. The walls of their cells have hardened to the point that when a low pressure comes in, the cells balloon up and pinch the nerves around them. They feel the discomfort. The body wasn't designed to do this, then how can it be fixed?

We can fix this with our little friend, Garlic. Garlic has the ability to soften the cell walls, thus allowing the pressure to equalize. When the cell walls are softened they can also get rid of toxins that are in each cell and take in the nutrition that it needs and wants. A lot of people use a product called MSM to do this, but Garlic already has organic Methylsufonylmethane in it.

O.K. so that is one of the many things that Garlic can do.

I had a friend ask me a few days ago, "What is the best herbal Antibiotic?" Of course my first reaction was to tell her Garlic but then I decided to see what Dr. James Duke had in his database on Antibiotics. According to him, Onion was the highest, another member of this wonderful family.

While I was in Dukes Database, I decided to see what other things Garlic could handle and I wasn't surprise. With over 200 components in these little bulbs, it packs a wallop. Some of the components had perfume as its ability and we have to admit that Garlic does emit a powerful smell but it is allowed to do that because of all its other abilities. I picked out a few that had many (not less than 5 and sometime many more) components working on this particular ability. What I found was that it is Antibacterial, Antidiabetic, Antiflu, Antiinflamatory, Antileukemic, Antioxident, Antiseptic, Antispasmodic, Antitumor, Antiviral, Cardioprotective, Chelates metals, is a fungicide, liver protective, perfumery, pesticide, and Vasodilator.

Now I have to tell a story about Garlic. I have a girlfriend who really believes in Garlic and felt that it kept her from getting sick. So she would eat a lot of it. Her business associates at work have asked her not to do this as they can smell it on her all the time. It got so bad that they suggested that she stay home until the smell was gone. She called me up and told me about this, wanting to know what would be just as Antiviral as Garlic. I suggested that she could come to my house and pick a bouquet of Lemon Balm. She could put these into a vase on her desk and nibble on the leaves until they were gone. Then she was always welcome to get another bouquet.

When one uses Garlic and it is opening the cell walls, it doesn't know that you don't want the skin cells opened. Its job is to open cell walls so the garlic smell permeates everything. The bad part is that like a smoker, the person eating Garlic doesn't notice this smell. They don't know that everything they wear smells like that too. Eating some Garlic will not create this problem, it is only a problem when one does a lot of it.

Garlic has been associated with a lot of folk lore. My guess is that even vampires don't like the smell.

Some of the properties that are in Garlic but not in large amounts are able to handle other things. They are Antialzheimeran, Antiarrhythmic, Antiasthmatic, Anticataract, Antilymphonic, Antiparkinsonian, Antistroke, and it even had a couple of its many properties that were AntiHIV. Plants really are designed to help us get and stay well.

It is my opinion that one should never take the same food all the time, and herbs are foods. One should vary what is being taken. I tell my classes that it wouldn't be a good idea to always have the same sandwich for every meal. We need to vary our diet so that the components that are in one food/herb are not duplicated all the time. We need a variety of components in our bodies, this way our body gets to choose what it wants and needs to stay healthy. The only exception to this would be when you are working on a specific problem. Let's say that you are working on the flu, and then you might want to use a lot of Garlic or whatever you have been using for this. Each food/herb gives the body choices of components to use for the benefit of keeping it in balance. The herbs/foods are in balance or they would not be healthy either.

There is a story about the European Plague. It goes something like this. It seems that people were dropping dead in the streets and no one wanted to move the bodies for fear of getting this plague. The police found that someone was touching these bodies and stealing all the jewelry and money on them. They finally caught the people doing this and told them that if they would tell how they could do this without getting sick, no charges would be brought. It seems that they had created a formula that they took. It was very high in Garlic. Dr. Christopher, one of my mentors created a formula based on this and called it his ANTIPLAGUE FORMULA.

I used this formula when I was treating my daughter. I didn't know what was wrong with her but she was very sick and had been for a week by the time she called me. She couldn't get her head off the pillow without a pounding headache. I gave her some peppermint tea and followed it up with a tablespoonful of Antiplague Formula. I did this every hour. (When treating a problem, herbs can be used every hour) By the fourth hour, she broke out with a major sweat; I bathed her and tucked her in for the rest of the night. I kept checking on her but she was sleeping so nicely that I didn't disturb her again. In the morning she was sitting next to my bed when I woke up. I asked if she wanted to lie down. She told me that it was so nice to be able to sit up and hold her head up and not feel sick but she thought that we would have to burn her nightie with its garlic smell. She also told me that the formula was "God Awful". I don't agree with her but it did the job.

Sometimes we have to bring out the big guns to heal and Garlic is one of my Big

Ginseng

Panax quinquefolia

This wasn't one of the herbs that I was going to include in this publication but I will do it as a tribute to my late sister, Donna.

I have Ginseng growing in my yard only because Donna knew someone who grew it in northern Wisconsin. She and I took a tour of his farm that had acres covered with wooden laths. The reason for this is that Ginseng grows in the woods. Wisconsin used to be all woods until it was ravaged like the rain forest. Ginseng likes shade. The grower told us that if a disease started in his field somewhere, all he had to do was remove some of the laths in that area and where ever the sun shone directly on the plants, they would die out, taking the disease with them. This way he could save most of his field. Every year he would plant a new acre. He always had 7 acres planted but at the end of the seventh year, that acre was harvested, dried, weighed and sold. Asians were the principal buyers.

So with seeds in hand, Donna and I set out to grow them. At first we grew them under some laths too but after a couple of years, they were moved to a wooded area where they still live. We harvested a couple of them a few years ago and made a tincture out of them. The rest are still growing. I like to go out in the late spring and see how many are still surviving. They wait until the trees start to leaf out and then come out of the ground. I have a sign up that says, "Donna's Ginseng."

Every year at least two of the plants grow a seed pod. They aren't really seed pods but more like five or six seeds clinging to the same area. When they get bright red I pull them off or they fall off

62

and I bury them. The next year I might find a couple of new plants in the area. The new babies have only three leaves as opposed to the mature plants that have five leaves. I have to be careful that I don't pull up the strawberry-like plants that look like they don't belong there.

Now let's find out why Ginseng is so wonderful. Some of the things that Ginseng is capable of doing are: being Antihistamine, Antitumor, Antibiotic, Antiinflammatory and a fungicide. It promotes the health of the liver and the heart along with slowing down coagulation time of the blood. It is also known to lower Blood pressure and works as a Vasodilator. According the Christopher Hobbs in his book THE GINSENGS – A USER'S GUIDE, Ginseng has the ability to lower blood sugar along with balancing out the adrenal output.

In Asia, Ginseng is used at a tonic for elderly people as it is supposed to increase the energy to major organs in the body. It balances the body out but also has a mildly sedative effect. One big plus is that it stimulates the brain and most elderly people like that effect.

It is also known that if taken regularly, it will improve vision so as you can see, it is a wonderful thing for the elderly. I think it is wonderful for anyone.

On the down side, it stimulates the uterus so it should be used with caution for pregnant women and women who tend to have excessive menses.

In spite of the coumarin-like effects, in Asia post-surgical patients are treated with a Ginseng mixture and recover faster than those without it.

Most of the Ginseng that is labeled Siberian Ginseng is really grown in Wisconsin but we won't tell anyone that. It is Wisconsin's major export.

Because the fields that have grown this cannot be used again for Ginseng, a few years ago farmers were looking for alternative plants to grow. I put out a suggestion that perhaps they could grow Echinacea. They only have to take down the laths as Echinacea likes sun and our cold winters.

Hawthorn

Crataegus oxyacantha

When Herbalist thinks of heart or heart problems, Hawthorn Berries come to mind and rightfully so, as you will soon see.

The Hawthorn tree usually grows from 15 to 30 feet in height. There are as many as 1000 species in North America. In my state I find the shorter variety. I find them in old farm fields as it is one of the first plants to start the change from the unused field back to forest. I find many people confusing the Buckthorn for Hawthorn and vice versa. There are two differences. One is the leaves of Hawthorn, which are similar to those of the apple family. The other is how the berries dangles from the branch, a lot like cherries. Neither of these are visible in the winter when people are chopping down trees with large thorns on them.

When you find a Hawthorn, you will understand its Latin name; "Crataegus" is Greek for hardness —of the wood. "Oxus" means sharp and "akantha" means a thorn. All are referring to the needle long thorns found on the branches. Also according to Mrs. Grieves in A MODERN HERBAL, the word "Haw" is an old word for hedge. This tree is also found as hedge filler in many areas.

The white flowers appear in May and turn into a bright red fruit that dries on the tree in the fall. This dried fruit is dark purple/red. It resembles a miniature stony apple. It has two large seeds in relationship to its pea-sized fruit. It should resemble the apple for it is another relative of the Rose family along with Apples, Apricots, Quince, Wild Cherries, Raspberries and Blackberries.

Now let me tell you how Hawthorn works on the heart muscle. The heart muscle needs calcium, potassium and magnesium. Hawthorn Berries are very high in the first two and sufficiently high in the third according to the constituents in Blake's Globalherb computer program.

Hawthorn has chromium.   It is said to lower bad cholesterol (LDL) and raise the good cholesterol (HDL). "Studies done by the Chinese state that Hawthorn Lowers cholesterol and triglycerides by improving excretion. It increases urination" according to Hanna Kroeger.

I have also heard that it keeps things from stagnating in the system; this could be a good way to keep the bowels moving?

A lot of my students are surprised to find out that the heart doesn't make the cholesterol.   This is made by the liver and the heart has to put up with this.   By the way, low cholesterol reading on a serum blood test doesn't mean that you have low cholesterol.   If all the cholesterol is attached to the walls of the veins and arteries, everything will look fine but your blood pressure will be high.   The heart just has to work harder to get the blood through your narrowing "pipes."   When there is high cholesterol or triglycerides, I tell my students to clean up the liver—a much better practice than using diuretics.   This can be handled with "Liver" herbs like Milk Thistle and Barberry.

Hawthorn also contains selenium and is recommended for weak hearts.   Selenium is very hard to find in our food because of the depleted farm soil but trees have the ability to put roots down 30 to 50 feet.   They don't depend on what we do to the top three feet of the soil.   When they want something to keep them healthy, they just extend a hair root and find what they need.   This is why everyone needs to be using some form of herb.   Our bodies need trace minerals. Herbs have trace minerals.   They are called trace minerals because we don't need a whole capsule of something like selenium.

Hawthorn, like its cousin the Apple, is very high in Vitamin C. When you combine Vitamin C with selenium, you have two of the most important Antioxidants in the nutritional world and they are said to protect against strokes. Vitamin C is very good at protecting the arteries against capillary breakage or leakage along with excessive clotting. It also helps to lower the cholesterol levels.

What we are doing with Hawthorn Berries is supplying the heart with all the elements that nourish it. In doing so we are allowing the heart to rebuild. I tell my students that you can't make a cake without flour and eggs in the house. When we nourish the body it does amazing things in the rebuilding area. With today's medicine we are in such a rush to transplant and drug the ill organ, when what we should be doing is supplying the body with what it needs to rebuild what we were originally given. Did you know that every organ can rebuild if 10% of the organ is healthy and you start to supply it with the right nutrition?

Hanna Kroeger, noted herbalist wrote, "Unlike digitalis, Hawthorn is not effective in correcting a complete failure as they don't contain the same compounds." Although she did use Blue Malva Tea to correct heart valve problems with much success.

The German equivalent to our FDA (Kommission E) published in their "*Monograph Notes*" that there were "No contra-indications from Hawthorn Berries. The German elderly used it as a tonic even without a heart condition" according to Kroeger.

There have been studies made in China showing a marked relief from angina attacks when using Hawthorn. Laboratory studies suggest that Hawthorn's action "May be created through the effects on the central nervous system. Oxygen levels increase in the heart," again according to Kroeger.

Other things that are seen as problems for the heart are, atherosclerotic (artery plaque), arteriosclerosis (hardening of the arteries), irregular heartbeats and palpitations, general tightness in the chest, difficult breathing and fatigue, all of which are treated in both China and Germany with the herb, Hawthorn.

Because of its ability to increase the force with which the heart contracts, it appears useful for congestive heart failure as suggested by Dr. Kim Vanderlinden in the *Health Counselor, Vol.7, No. 4.*

Dr. Shen, a Chinese herbalist, whom I met on the Internet, suggests Chinese sage (Dan Shen) 9gm, Safflower (Hong Hua) 9gm, Pseudoginseng root (San Qi) 3 gms and Chinese Licorice root (Zhi gan Cao) 6 gms. Slow boil the herbs in 4 cups of water for 40 minutes. Drink twice a day along with Hawthorne and Ginseng for "Remarkable recovery from by-pass surgery."

In my herbal classes, my students enjoy learning how to make a tonic and the one we make is a Hawthorn Berry Tonic. This is made by soaking the dried berries, then simmering them for 20 to 30 minutes, strain and return the liquid to a cleaned kettle. We add to this, raw sugar (SUCANAT), cool and bottle it. This is good for many months in the refrigerator as the sugar is a preservative and raw sugar add properties such as vitamins and mineral also. I like to add some Black Cherry Juice Concentrate for flavor but Hawthorn has a nice taste of its own.

While making the tonic, we are struck by its dark red/purple color. This is the compound known as flavonoids. Hawthorn Berries have a large amount of this substance which is said to balance the body's hormones. "Flavonoids work with Vitamin C (Hawthorn being high in Vitamin C) to build bones, collagen, tendons, capillaries and strong teeth according to Kroger. Sounds like additional bonuses?

Flavonoids made the news a while ago when some French study came out exclaiming that a glass of red wine daily would help one to have a healthy heart. It is the purple skin in the grape that is loaded with Flavonoids as are the other members of the Rose family, namely the dark-skinned berries.

Hawthorn Berry Tonic is normally taken daily over time to reap the results that have been mentioned here, so it surprised me when one person told me of experiencing pain periodically in the upper left arm and by taking a dose of Hawthorn Tonic, was relieved within the hour.

There are many other herbs that affect the heart but none quite as effective yet mild and safe as Hawthorn.

Ԉorsetail Grass

Equisetum arvense

I grew up on a lake in upper Wisconsin, just the kind of place that Horsetail grass loves. It has an affinity for having wet feet and it does that by being next to a lake, stream, or pond.

Horsetail grass grew all over our yard. As kids we would pull it up and because it grows in segments, looks green, and is skinny we called it snake grass. I don't think I realized that there are two kinds, male and female because to a kid they all looked alike.

The male looks like a green hollow pencil, straight and tall with pull-apart divisions and a bulbous head on the top. The female has whorls of tiny branches at each of the divisions on the stem. These plants are rather rough and hard due to their high mineral content. We would chew on them like a straw.

In one book that I read, it talked about this plant being a dinosaur. That at one time it grew very large like a tree. In our yard it grew less than a foot tall. I have seen taller ones.

It wasn't until I start studying plants that I realized this plaything from my childhood had value. Isn't that the way it is with all of us. We don't understand what is right in our own back yards.

Dr. Christopher talked about that. One of the things that he said was to "eat under your own fig tree." We need to learn what lives around us and how to use it not only as medicine but as food. Hey, I keep saying that they are interchangeable. We have been taught to eat a lot of foods to sustain our bodies. I even was required to do a menu for my degree to see how much I would have to eat to get the Recommended Daily Allowance of everything. I don't think we need to eat that much. I think if we are getting the "right stuff" we don't need all of what is required by the government studies. We just really need a variety.

Horsetail grass is loaded with silica. So who cares about that? Silica is not something that is required by the RDA, but unless you have it in your body, any calcium coming in your direction will not be utilized. According to Dr. Christopher, "As explained in the book Biological Transmutations, The silica in horsetail grass converts to calcium, and the other herbs work in close conjunction with this master calcium herb." (See The Mucusless Diet by Dr. Christopher.)

David Christopher said that bones heal faster when there is a higher amount of silica in the blood than calcium.

The way that the Native Americans used this plant was to gather them together and use them to scrub things. It is the hardness of this plant that they used.

The next time you are near water, look around and see if Horsetail lives in that area.

Ꮒyssop
Ꮒyssopus officinalis

Hyssop is a small shrub like plant that is a member of the mint family. It tends to grow about 1 to 2 feet high with square stems like its cousins. The three varieties with Purple/blue, red or white flowers in whorls give the plant family away. The plants flower from June to October and make a very nice border plant. Hyssop has been naturalized in the United States having been brought here from Southern Europe. The hot spicy smell makes this a most agreeable plant. Its taste is somewhat bitter. These plants require cutting occasionally, but do not need much more attention according to Mrs. Grieve in her A MODERN HERBAL books.

Hyssop is spoken of in the Bible (Psalms 51:7) in connection with cleansing and purifying the body. "Purge me with Hyssop, and I shall be clean". Mrs. Grieve suggested that the Hebrew plant called "Ezeb" has been translated "Hyssop" and this is said to have grown out of the walls of the temple. According to her it is quite possible that the name is applied to several plants of similar properties.

The Greeks called it Hyssopos as a name of a Holy herb, because it was used to clean sacred places. It seems that evil spirits hated it. I have used this plant to clear/clean negative energies out of my home. I even gave cuttings away to people that need to clean negative energies from their living and working spaces.

I have found it will change an unhappy person into someone who can be dealt with. Hyssop was brought into a room where a blind person had become very cranky and was crying all the time. She was not aware that the Hyssop was there but it seemed to calm her down and she became herself again.

70

Hyssop is a most widely used purification herb in magic. It is added to baths in sachets, infused or sprinkled on objects or persons to cleanse them, and hung up in homes to purge them of evil and negativity, according to the Cunningham's Encyclopedia of Magical Herbs.

The tops and leaves are used in teas and tinctures and are valuable for asthma, colds, grippe and all chest afflictions along with shortness of breath. It is also an excellent blood regulator as it increases the circulation of the blood and reduces blood pressure. It is a great tonic for mucus tissue of both the respiratory and the gastrointestinal tracts in all weakened conditions. "Serviceable in connection with hygienic herbs, scrofula, gravel, various stomach complaints, jaundice, dropsy, spleen malfunctions. Has been used in herbal preparations for epilepsy. It has been used as a gargle with sage for sore throats." All according to Alma Hutchens in her book, INDIAN HERBALOGY OF NORTH AMERICA.

Hutchens also sights Plants Used Against Cancer, A Survey by Hartwell, for its mention as being used against sclerosis of the liver and tumors.

Medicinally it has been used as an expectorant, diaphoretic, stimulant and carminative. The healing virtues of the plant are due to the volatile oils. It has been used as a warm infusion mixed with horehound. Hyssop tea is a grateful drink for toning feeble stomachs, being brewed with the green tops. The leaves can be used externally for relief of muscular rheumatism and for bruises and discolored contusions. The bruised green herb will heal cuts promptly. Hyssop has been used in baths as part of the cure for rheumatism.

The flower-tops have also been used as a kitchen herb in salads and broths. If I remember right, Grieves mentioned that any household with an illness should include stews and soups with Hyssop tops for the health of the family. Herbs are food, enjoy.

Lamb's Quarters

Chenopodium album

Lamb's Quarters not to be confused with Lamb's Ears, is this little weed often called Pigweed.

It is the first thing that we pull out of our gardens when weeding. No one I knows cultivates it as it has so little appeal. There is only green; green leaves, green flowers, and green seeds. I have seen it growing up to 4 feet tall and taking over an area of the garden. It grows mostly where the soil has been disturbed, as in gardens or even new construction.

It has been used as a food for a long time as it is a cousin to Spinach. When the plants are less than 10 inches high they are tender and can be cooked as a pot herb. They have the taste of pea pods. They are very high in Vitamin C, Vitamin A, thiamin, riboflavin and niacin.

What I am finding in Duke's Database states that this plant has some things in it that are: Anticataract, Antiasthmatic, Antimalarial, Antidiabetic, Antieczemic, Antiparkinsonian, and Antipapillomic (This last one is the virus that they are giving young girls a vaccine for so that they can be "one less". There are 72 papillomas and the shot takes care of only four of them. Even men can get this virus.) Hey, this plant isn't going to do it all but if you nibble on a leaf here and there; it sure gives the body more than what we are getting in our food supply.

According to Dr. Christopher it is a very good source of much usable calcium. I eat the leaves raw while I am in the yard or put them into a salad with tomatoes, celery, purslane, chickweed and add any dressing, my favorite being oil and vinegar. This is a great way to get my calcium with lots of flavors.

The American Indians used the leaves to treat stomachaches and prevent scurvy. Using the cold tea is known to check diarrhea. A leaf poultice is great for burns. As a folk remedy Lamb's Quarters is used for vitiligo, a skin disorder where the pigment is not present.

The next time you see this plant, taste a leaf, I think you will like it.

Marshmallow

Althaea officinalis

The Malva family is extensive as are most families but this family has a history of cleaning up "old wounds". One member of this family is the Marshmallow. I have used Marshmallow Root to clean up major situations so I call it one of my "big Guns" as it does what it says it will do. (As you read this book you will find that I have a several "Big Guns" that I can count on.)

Dr. John Christopher referred to this plant when he explained how to "cure" gangrene. Actually he was referring to a cousin of Marshmallow called Common Malva and it grows everywhere. As a small plant, it is found growing around outbuildings and in gardens. I find that it invades my front gardens and has to be pulled out all the time. Another name for Common Malva is "Cheese its" as the seed pods look like cheese rounds. Dr. Christopher mentioned that Malvas are effective demulcents. (Having mucilaginous properties that are soothing and will remove rough skin, dandruff and dry scabs anywhere on the body.)

Christopher's plan to cure gangrene is to gather a handful of the whole plant of Common Malva and put it into a bucket. Fill this with water as hot as healthy skin can stand. Then put the gangrenous body part into this for 20 minutes. After that period of time transfer the limb to cool water for 10 minutes. Make another batch of the hot Malva tea and put the limb back into this for 20 minutes. Continue this process all day until ready for bed. The next day start all over. He suggested that within a couple of days you will see results. This is obviously not a one-person job.

I was on vacation when my sister called and told me what was happening to our Mother. I suggested a variation of this program as the one foot and leg that was black and had two ulcerated sores on the foot. After putting Slippery Elm on the ulcerated sores, Betty wrapped Mom's leg and foot with cotton strips and kept the strips wet with a tea made of Marshmallow Root. The sores scabbed over and the leg turned purple with pink strips within four days. Within a week, the scabs were still there but the leg and foot turned baby pink. While doing something like this one needs to have the Marshmallow working on the inside as well as the outside. Teas and Capsules are great for this.

This was done not without problems. Mom's caregiver wanted to turn us into the health department for not getting proper care for our Mother. We asked her to give us two weeks and then she would be welcome to do that. What would they have done for Mother? They would have removed her leg at the knee. Can you believe that we are still in the dark ages? My husband's uncle had this same problem and they removed first his toes and then his leg.

Herbs were given to us by GOD. They work wonders if we know how to use them.

Recently I bought a bottle of Marshmallow capsules for myself. I had a burning sensation in my esophagus which could have been acid reflux and I knew that Marshmallow would handle this in a breeze. I put a capsule in my mouth and flooded it with water. When the capsule opened, I swallowed a little at a time to allow enough herb in contact with the skin on the way down. Due to it mucilaginous properties, it tends to attach to the walls of the esophagus and starts the healing immediately.

The bottle that I bought said, "It has been speculated that a confection made of marshmallow inspired our modern-day candy, even though it does not actually contain the herb." That will give you an idea of how it tasted in my mouth.

I had a call from a lady who had returned from Las Vegas. She had gone to her doctor to find out how to get rid of the diarrhea that she had since her return. After using the doctor's medicine for this for a couple of weeks and still having diarrhea, she called to see what I would suggest. I mentioned that Marshmallow Capsules might be helpful. She then told me that she would get some and try it as soon as the medicine ran out. I am not a doctor and not allowed to prescribe for anyone but I suggested that she start taking the Marshmallow Capsules that night and see if it made a difference. Not to take her medicine for the rest of that day but she could start again tomorrow if necessary. She called the next day and couldn't believe that her diarrhea had stopped after only taking 3 of the capsules of Marshmallow Root. I told her to continue taking the Marshmallow for another few days to clean up any residue problem.

Another cousin in the Malva family is the Hollyhock. Like all members of this family, Hollyhock leaves crushed and soaked can be used as a poultice on bed sores and healing happens more quickly than with the ointments that are presently used to protect these areas. Hollyhock leaves contain the nourishment required for rebuilding the skin.

The root of the Mallow has been used again tuberculosis as it is said to have Antiinflammatory properties and be a mild astringent. Dr. Varro Tyler mentioned that the Kommission E (the German FDA) "has declared them all (the Mallows or Malvas) to be good for things like coughs and bronchitis."

Both Steven Foster and James Duke mention that common Mallow Tea has been used for angina. This doesn't surprise me. Hanna Kroeger use Blue Malva flowers to rebuild heart valves. Her formula was, "1 cup twice daily for 6 weeks to rebuild heart valves." I suggested four drops of this tea for a new born that needed a new heart valve, four times a day. About a week later they called to tell me that they had to stop doing this. The child who had been limp as a dishrag was now so playful that he didn't want to sleep...I suggested cutting it back to four drops twice in the early part of the day. The parents told me that the child never had surgery as the doctors felt that he had out grown the problem. (Aren't these God given things wonderful?)

We had an old cat that was always hungry and never seemed to keep anything down for long. I mixed some Marshmallow root into her food and she didn't seem to be meowing (crying) all the time.

Our animals can use herbs just like we do. The dosage is different as we gear to the size of the animal.

Cats would only get one-fourth of a human dose.

Small Dogs would get a half of a human dose.

Large dogs could have a full human dosage as would horses.

Two weeks ago a friend called to tell me that she was having a urinary tract infection (UTI) She told me what she was using herbally and that it was working from time to time but it didn't clear up. I told her that I would do some research and get back to her. I checked Dr. James Duke's Database and found that the third product down on the list for urinary tract infections was Marshmallow. They have a certain constituent that "hits" UTIs. I didn't recognize the top two herbs. She said that she would try that. I got an email from her and it is gone. Sometimes these herbs amaze even me as I am always learning. I would not have thought to use Marshmallow for this but it works.

Even the leaves of the Malvas when bruised will take away the pain, redness and swelling of insect stings.

Keep this "Big Gun" ready for anything in your health department.

Lemon Balm
Melissa officinalis

In my garden I have this mild mint that has a lemon taste to the leaves. She looks so innocent but just wait until I tell you about her; it will knock your socks off.

First I have to tell you about her name. It is an abbreviation of the Latin Melossophyllum, meaning bee plant. According to Simon & Schuster's Guide to Herbs and Spices, it was thought that if you rubbed the branches of Melissa over new hives, it would attract swarms of bees to start a new colony.

Lemon Balm originally came from Europe and has been naturalized in my area. These mints have a way of finding their own home wherever they are.

The leaves are opposite heart-shaped with "dentate-crenate" margins, which means that it has scalloped edges similar to its cousin, Catnip. On tasting the leaves you can tell the difference. The leaves are full of oil-bearing glands that give off a wonderful lemon taste/smell. This is due to the presence of ethereal oils, notably citral and citronellal. Citronellal being the oil that is widely used to repel bugs, this could tell you of one of the many great things for which you can use Melissa.

According to what I have read about this plant, one should replace the plants every five years, but in my garden it seems that they do this all by themselves. I only have to remove the older ones and I have more than enough two-foot high Lemon Balm plants.

The best time to harvest the leaves is just before, or at the time that flowers start to appear. I have found when you need the plant is really the best time to harvest. I always thank her for the leaves that I take, from spring until fall.

One of the experts on this plant is Dr. Varro E. Tyler, a Professor of Pharmacognosy at Purdue University. I decided to see what he had to say about this lovely garden plant in his book HERBS OF CHOICE. The first thing that I learned from him was that people have been using Lemon Balm for 20 centuries. There must be something important about it. He mentioned that it was a calming herb. It also has Antibacterial properties. Now I am really excited.

This calmative effect that he speaks about is one of many uses. I like to cut some Melissa and stuff it into a clean sock, then dump the sock into my bath tub and I get to soak in a Lemon Balm tea. The whole tub is my tea cup. It is so relaxing that it is even suitable for small children. When taking a "Tub Tea" it is helpful to drink a cup of it also. (Not what is in the tub but a cup of Melissa Tea made before you hop in.) This allows the active ingredients to help from the inside also and Melissa does just that. Her properties tend to open the skin pores and allow the toxins in the body to exit while calming the whole body surface.

Once after going to get a massage from a "deep-muscle" masseuse, I went home with the idea that I needed to relax (For those of you who have never had a "Deep-muscle" massage; when you are done you know where every body part is; as they are all telling you that they have been moved about.) I ran a bath and decided that I would put Lemon Balm in the water. I cut two bundles and tied them together. As I was sitting in the water, I noticed that it was turning black. The massage oil was being pulled out into the bath water and the chemical reaction turned the water "Nylon stocking" black. I could still see through it but what a strange reaction.

Dr. Tyler also mentioned that, "In 1978 it was first demonstrated to have Antiviral activity. The caffeic acid oxidation product is said to inhibit not only Herpes simplex type 1 virus, which causes cold sores, but the Herpes simplex type 2 virus, which causes genital lesions " He mentioned that in Europe "they are currently marketing a pharmaceutical product for use on both Herpes type 1 and type 2 using the concentrated extract of Melissa. " He mentioned that no side effects having been reported with this plant and its extracts.

In view of that I must add that recently I read that Herpes Simples Virus Type 1 is the major cause of the protein plaque that creates Alzheimer's. (I cannot confirm this but thought that the information was worth including here.)

Everyone knows how it feels to be getting a cold sore on the lips, the tingling feeling. I was under a lot of stress and could feel that feeling coming on so I put a dropperful of Melissa tincture in my mouth and sucked in the area that was giving me that tingly feeling. In essence, I was bathing that area with this tincture. I did this three times one day and never did get the cold sore.

It seems that this little mint is most powerful with Antiviral properties and mild enough for children. How silly I was just using it as a relaxing bath when it can do so much more.

A friend of mine was trying to get and stay healthy by eating Garlic all the time. After a while her co-workers told her that if she was going to continue to eat Garlic, not to come to work. So she called me all upset and wanted to know what she could do as she felt that Garlic was really helping her. I told her to come over to my house and pick a bouquet of Lemon Balm from my garden. These could be placed in a vase on her desk and she can continue to eat the leaves until the bouquet is gone; then she could come back to pick another bouquet. She would have something so Antiviral and so tasty and so lemony that no one could complain.

At our house, dried Lemon Balm is used over broiled fish to give it a little lemon flavor and a lot of antiviral, which my family doesn't have to know about. It can be added to soups, stews and salads.

The next time you find yourself facing a Lemon Balm plant, give her the respect that she deserves. She might look like just one of the "nice little" mints but she is powerful.

CDotherwort

Leonurus cardiaca

This morning my body told me to talk about Motherwort. I woke up with tightness in my chest. This is not unusual as my family has a history of heart problems. I usually don't do anything about this until my left arm starts to bother me but today my body was talking to me. So after getting out of bed, I headed for my Motherwort tincture. After taking 15 drops of this tincture and washing it down with water, I feel much better, herbs always amaze me.

Many people have written about Motherwort as improving several aspects of coronary health by improving circulation and strengthen the muscles ability to function. It will calm palpitations and normalize heart function

Motherwort is a member of the mint family and found growing wild in my back yard. It has the most distinctive leaves of all the mints. When the plant first comes up, its leaves have almost a geranium type look to them. (This is why when I go to clean up the gardens in the spring; I have to leave some of the plants that I can't identify because they might just turn out to be someone special.) As this plant starts growing up from the middle of this rosette of leaves, the leaves change and have a three-fingered look; with the middle part being the longest. Once you have seen these leaves, you will always be able to identify this plant. Like all mints, the flowers are formed in whorls on the top of this stalk.

Most people think of the mint family as little sweet tasting plants such as Peppermint or Spearmint but the family is extensive and some have a way of packing a punch.

Dr. James Duke has identified almost 50 constituents in Motherwort. Some of which have the ability to be: Antitumor, Antioxidant, Antibacterial, Antiviral and Antiarrhythmic. Combined with the rest of the properties in this herb, they have the ability to assist our bodies in marvelous ways and all these constituents are organic.

Why is organic so great? Because we are organic beings so why would we put chemicals that are made from petroleum or rocks into our bodies? One of the great things about using herbs is that they contain many things making them good for handling a lot of different areas.

With nick names like "heart gold", " heart heal", "heart wort" and "heart herb", one would think that this was just a cardiac herb but Motherwort tends to handle problems in other organs. It will help the eyes, gall bladder, the nervous system and the generative organs.

In regard to the generative organs (after all it is called Motherwort) It is great at assisting with delayed menses or stopped menses and even postpartum depression. It would also be helpful for cramps and other fertility issues.

Mullein

Verbascum thapsus

In March I transplanted a second year Mullein into my yard. Mullein is a biennial plant. Last year I had 5 second-year plants in the front yard. These five to seven foot soft giants dominated my west berm where they allowed me to harvest their leaves. When mature the lower leaves are eighteen to twenty four inches long. They are soft and fuzzy, giving this plant the nick name of "camper's toilet paper." The leaves give way to flowers about three feet off the ground, leaving the top three to four feet looking like a pillar of tiny yellow flowers. The flowers tell us about their family as they belong to the snapdragon family (Scrophulariaceae). The first-year plant is a rosette of large, soft leaves, which is not to be confused with Lamb's ears that have a more upright, pointed leaf.

According to one herbal author, Mullein is a household herb that has been used a very long time. The leaf tea has been used for asthma, bronchitis and all kinds of lung afflictions. In the area of lungs, American Indians would smoke mullein to heal the lungs. They also used this tea as a throat gargle, for toothaches and for washing open sores. The flower tea can be used to relieve pain, induce sleep and (in large doses) as a laxative. Some writers even felt that the fresh crushed flowers would remove warts.

I have read where the leaves or flowers when made into a tea were helpful for kidneys.

I have used the leaves as a poultice for skin sores but due to the leaf hairs it is best to make the poultice and encase it in a cloth when put next to the skin. The woolly leaves can be used as an emergency bandage while in the wilderness.

83

My very personal experience with Mullein started when I was told by one of my teachers, "If an organ is dead, it will decay and poison the body. Surgery will be need. If it isn't dead, heal it!"

I took that to heart. I had been taking Synthyroid for 15 years. I also had been told by the medical community that I would need to take this for the rest of my life. My thyroid wasn't dead, just not working. How was I going to heal it?

In one of Dr. John Christopher's lectures, he mentions that 3 parts of Mullein and one part of Lobelia heals glands. He was talking about the lymph system at the time. He created this formula for the purpose of healing glands. My thyroid is a gland so I just had to try this.

I decided to see what would happen if I took one Synthyroid tables and one Mullein and Lobelia capsule a day. I did this for forty days as it sounded like a good time period to start some healing. I wondered how these herbs would know which gland to help first. Maybe all my glands needed healing? Dr. Christopher did say that Lobelia, being a "thinking herb" would direct it to the place most needing help.

Being a person of faith, I set off on my adventure but in the back of my mind I worked out Plan B. (Always have a plan B.) How will I know if it has healed? I remembered the enlargements in the throat area and the headaches from my jaw to the top of my head before Synthroid. If these symptoms returned I would retreat back to my "Pills". So my "pills" were hidden in one of my dresser drawers, just in case.

I must remind the reader that healing without feeding is futile. The thyroid needs iodine to function. Along with the chemical pills and herbal capsules, I was feeding the thyroid organic iodine. Mullein and Lobelia will not do this. Organic iodine is found in kelp and black walnut hulls. I chose to take one kelp capsule a day during this period.

In Hanna Kroeger's book, GOD HELPS THOSE THAT HELP THEMSELVES, I learned that Sodium Fluoride is detrimental to the thyroid. It was a good time to find a new toothpaste. I learned that the body need calcium fluoride to stay healthy **not** sodium fluoride.

Sodium Fluoride has been used to rid mice from Granaries. It is a lot more poisonous than people think. The dental community knows that Fluoride is good for the body but it isn't Sodium-Fluoride but

Calcium Fluoride that the body can use. Hanna has a lot of information on this in her books.

All of this happened in the early 1990's. After my experiment, I used The Mullein and Lobelia caps on a daily basis for a while. After a few months, I only took them once a week. Now I do it as needed. I did have a problem about three months into this program and instead of remembering my "Pills", I doubled up on the Mullein and Lobelia. Within a day, the enlargement and the headache was gone. When I find myself getting tired more than usual, I know that it is a thyroid problem. Then it is time to work on that area of my body again.

A cousin called me because she had a thyroid problem and wanted to get off her "pills" too. I told her what I did and she did the program. After some time she called to tell me that her throat was giving her a problem. I suggested making a poultice out of the Mullein and Lobelia Capsules and wrapping it around her throat, then climbing into a hot tub while drinking some tea made out of these capsules. She thanked me for the suggestion and when I didn't hear from her for a few days, I contacted her. I asked how she was and she acted like she didn't know what I was talking about. Why? Because she expected this to work; I was just suggesting it and hoping it would work.

Last year I had an accident and bruised a knee. The chiropractor told me that the end of the leg bone was saturated with blood like a sponge. That is why I had trouble walking on it. I knew that I was going to have to work on the lymph system to get this old, dried-up blood out so the leg could heal. It was back to my Mullein and Lobelia again. Lobelia would know where I needed the Mullein the most. This time I didn't need the Kelp.

Being able to help myself to good health is wonderful.

In truth, herbs do not heal but furnish the area with all the building blocks needed to heal. They also clean out toxins and unneeded properties allowing the cells to regenerate according to God's plan (DNA/RNA)

Learning about herbs is a lifelong study with 200,000 medicinal herbs and all of them can be used for so many things. It is nice to find a few friends that one can count on like Mullein

Oak

Quercus alba

Oak, Oak, the Mighty Oak. How many poems have been written about, "The Mighty Oak?" How many stories revolve around "The Mighty Oak?" The magic of Oak is not just for legends; "the Mighty Oak" is for health as well.

It is the inner bark of the oak that we use mainly for health. Oak Bark is astringent, antiseptic, and tonic. These are the properties that Dr. John Christopher of the School of Natural Healing used to tighten teeth. He put a strip of the inner bark of the Oak between the teeth and gums and left it there. Not only did this tighten the teeth but the gums absorbed nutrition from the bark. (We are aware that nutrition can be absorbed through the skin.) He suggested that if this was done regularly, the gums would not recede. He stated that receding gums is not an old age problem as we have been lead to believe but the lack of nutrition to this area.

As for the antiseptic properties, Dr. Christopher felt that one could use a wash of Oak Bark tea along with the strips of bark or capsules to correct pyorrhea.

He also mentioned in one of his lectures about the high content of absorbable Calcium in Oak Bark. This is why he put it in his "Complete Tissue (Bones, Flesh and Cartilage) formula". All plants have calcium. They build with it. The wood in your house is made from their calcium deposits and the other minerals that have been in them when they were alive. Every time you eat a plant, you are taking in calcium. If you have a diet that consists of fruits, vegetables, grains, nuts and seeds, you are getting calcium. We really get all the calcium that we need in our diet if we are eating properly but we lose so much due to an improper diet of sugar and having our bodies in the condition where they aren't able to utilize or absorb the nutrition that is available.

Oak Bark is designed to utilize the calcium that it contains using all the trace minerals that are in it. Dr. Christopher knew that we were not getting all these trace minerals, so he created an "Herbal Calcium Formula" that is made up of Horsetail grass, Oat straw, Nettle and Lobelia herb to support mineral absorption.

He talked about needing whole foods containing all these trace minerals and not just taking calcium tablets that are grounded up sea shells or mined rocks. Plant calcium is cell sized and can be used by the body. Calcium tablets tells the body that here is some needed calcium but it is too big for the body's cells so the body parks it in joints until it can break it down and use it. Minerals need acid to be broken down and the body works best in an alkaline range.

I decided to find out how to put more calcium in my body with some of these plants. Over the past few years I have changed my diet to limit my intake of sugar. According to Dr. Christopher, sugar pulls calcium out of the body. I found that when I had some sugar (Birthday Cake, etc.) I would have leg cramps during the night. I knew that meant a calcium loss. So after any intake of sugar, I would supplement my body with a couple cups of Oak Bark tea or some capsules with Oak Bark in them and like magic, I didn't have leg-cramps.

A couple of books that I have read mention that oak bark has a bitter taste. I have not found this to be true. I remember one time while I was buying some bulk Oak Bark at Outpost Natural Foods, a lady asked me what it tasted like. I was stumped for a little while and then it came to me. It tastes like sawdust. This took me back to my childhood when my sisters and I used sawdust as pretend food in our doll house. (A rather pleasant memory.)

The useful properties of Oak Bark can be extracted easily in both water and spirits.

This tea is great at correcting mucus situations in the body, thus it is helpful for sinus congestion and postnasal drip, etc. Oak

Bark tea can also be applied to any open sore and wrapped. This reduces swelling.

Due to its astringent properties, the tea can also be used in sitz baths for hemorrhoids and prolapsed rectum. It stops bleeding both externally and internally.

Dr. Christopher talked about using Oak Bark as a paint on varicose veins. He mentioned that one could simmer the bark in water while reducing the water and then adding more bark until it was the consistency of lacquer. This could be painted on the legs or where ever needed and the body would use it to handled the problems. This would be repeated as often as it was absorbed.

Many Oak trees create galls or growths to deal with insects that bother them. These galls are super high in astringent properties and can be used where the skin needs to be tightened. A tincture of oak galls can be used to arrest bleeding from nose bleeds to hemorrhoids. An infusion is wonderful as a gargle to relax the throat and for inflamed tonsils.

Oak Bark is known to expel worms and parasites from the body. It is also know to be antiviral and antioxidant.

Herbalists have used all parts of the oak from the acorn to the leaves for various purposes.

American Indians used the fruit of the tree as food. By rinsing the tannins out of the pulped acorns with many rinses, it was a ready food. They also would take a hunk of bark and put the inner bark next to a wound, then wrap the area and continue on their way. This allowed the inner bark to start the healing. According to Dr. James Duke, Oak Bark is very high in Antibacterial properties and quite high in Antiinflammatory properties, perfect for starting the healing process.

As you can see "The Mighty Oak" has earned its reputation as a MIGHTY HEALER.

Peppermint
Mentha piperita

Most people know about Peppermint because it has been put in everything from candy to candles. I want to tell you what Peppermint can do for your body.

Because of its many properties, it does many jobs. One of them is to be a stimulant, let's start with that and talk about Peppermint's very high vibration. This means that compared to most other plants, Peppermint will create more benefits than a lot of herbs. It is included in a lot of formulas, perhaps to make them work harder? It tends to raise the level of the bodies pH to an alkaline state. (This is very good because the body is happier when it is slightly alkaline as opposed to acid. Most of the foods that we eat such as meat, dairy, and "dead" foods tend to be acid.) Having something that can adjust the pH before we even get started is wonderful.

I find that giving someone a cup of Peppermint tea before I start them on a program of herbs is like jump starting a car. The body is perked up and ready to do some work for me. As a stimulant, Peppermint gets things moving faster to handle what needs to be done.

Peppermint is the most pungent in the mint family. At the Celestial Seasonings Tea Company in Boulder Colorado, Peppermint has its own store room as it would adulterate the other teas and tea combination in the main warehouse.

More of the exciting stuff in this same herb are the properties that are sedative, nervine and Antispasmodic in their abilities. Peppermint has a calming effect on most people, even children. It can be used to soothe and make one sleepy. As a nervine, it will help rebuild nerve cells and as an antispasmodic, it is great for stomach problems, while aiding with digestion.

When I lived in the Los Angeles area, I met a lady from England. She told me that when people wanted to lose weight, they would drink Peppermint tea. It has a wonderful refreshing taste without any sweeteners added; it also cleans and tones the entire body.

My mentors have mentioned that one should never boil an herb that is as volatile as Peppermint. A lot of its healing is done with the oils in this plant. The best way to use Peppermint is as a tea by pouring hot water over the leaves that have already been put into a cup. Cover the cup and allow steeping for 10 min. Although I prefer chewing on a leaf when I am in my garden.

Peppermint oil is used a lot in aroma therapy. So I want to tell you about oils. It takes 50 pounds of most plant materials to make 1/2 oz of pure oil from a plant. When using oils it is recommended to put them in a carrier oil. Talk to an aromatherapist if this is the route that you choose to go.

Pure Peppermint oil can be toxic when used in large amounts as written up by I. Thorup in his paper called Toxicol. It seems that he did research on this oil and found that it would create lesions in the brain of rats when used in large amount. He mentioned that humans couldn't take enough oil internally to create this problem.

David Christopher, director of the School of Natural Healing talked about some studies like the one above by I. Thorup and how they test. He said that they give lab rats the equivalent of feeding a human one hundred times what a real human would eat. The lab rat is taking in 100 or more times its body weight in whatever they are testing and when the animal gets cancer, they then decide that this substance is toxic. Perhaps our standards of testing products need a change?

I have been reading THE HEALING POWER OF HERBS by Michael T. Murray N.D. and was surprised to learn that Peppermint has Antiviral activity. Dr. Murray mentioned that Peppermint inhibits growths of "Newcastle Disease virus, Herpes simplex virus and vaccine virus." He mentioned that the properties most likely to do this can be found in a simple tea.

Do you think that the healing of virus or bacteria could take place because of the energy in this plant? This subject is the basis of Dr. Theodore A. Baroody's book , ALKALIZE OR DIE.

Most people agree that the active ingredient is the menthol but with about 240 components in this one plant, it is hard to pin one thing down. Chemists want to take things apart to find out what does what but when you find a plant like Peppermint and know all the great things that it can do in just a cup of tea, it is time to sit back, relax and enjoy a wholesome healing.

Plantain

Plantago major

We are going to talk about what was an illegal substance. No, I'm not talking about Cocaine or Marijuana. I am going to discuss a weed called Plantain or Plantago major, not to be confused with the Plantain that looks like bananas.

This little weed grows in every yard that hasn't been sprayed. For those of you who are fussy about your yard, the bad thing about Plantain is that it's wide leaves tend to spread out and when the plant is pulled out by its single root, it leaves a large bare spot about the size of a dinner plate. In my state, we mostly find the wide leaf variety but there is a narrow leaf variety also.

The spoon-shaped wide leaves are very identifiable by the fact that the leaf stem is an extension of the leaf. Its seeds are on a spike that grows 5 to 10 inches up from the center of this plant. These seeds are used as a laxative (Psyllium).

Before I tell you about the "miracles" this little plant does, let's go back to why it was illegal. In 1997 a company called RISE AND SHINE from the Northwest United States bought some Plantain and received Fox Glove by mistake. According to the source of this information, *A Healthier You*, which is a newsletter put out by David Christopher M.H., It was caught before anyone got hurt (Fox Glove is the source of Digitalis which affects the heart muscle.) The Food and Drug Administration decided that there was a big problem and in 1997 banned Plantain. Did they ban Fox Glove? According to David, they did not.

A few years ago the FDA banned Chaparral and sprayed large sections of desert where it grew. Chaparral is very effective as a blood cleanser, so much so that it is used with success for certain cancers. Why is this being mentioned here, because the FDA seems to have made incorrect decisions. Are they still making them?

Now, why is Plantain so exciting to herbalist? First, because it is very safe! It is so safe that it can be eaten like lettuce. Also, because it is the very best herb at drawing poisons out of the body. With a bug bite or sting, the crushed leaf of the Plantain will draw the poison, along with the stinger out promptly.

At a rally being held at an organic farm that I was attending, a couple of workers came running up to me telling me that there was a problem. It seems that one of the other guests had put a soda can down and when he went to drink it, he swallowed a bee. They wanted to see if there was something that could be done. I talked to the man and it seemed that he had been stung in the esophagus. So we went to the garden and pulled up some plantain. I told him to chew on the leaves but only swallow the juice. While he was doing that, I got some Cayenne and water ready. After chewing on a few leaves and spitting them out, I had him drink the Cayenne water. This did not make him happy. My next thing was to tell him that if at any time he was having trouble taking a deep breath or swallowing, he was to go to the local hospital about 5 miles away. I kept an eye on this man for the rest of the time that I was there and he didn't seem to be in a hurry to leave. His family was playing around having a lot of fun.

A couple of weeks later, I asked the manager of the organic farm if he knew what had happened to that man. He said that he didn't know but gave me a phone number. I called and asked the man what had happened. He was so angry over the phone. He told me how terrible it was that I gave him the cayenne water as his throat burned all afternoon. I told him that I was sorry to hear that but I was smiling while I said this. After hanging up I knew that this man didn't have a clue how dangerous this could have been. The Plantain had pulled some of the toxin out of the area and the cayenne drew the blood to this area to clean up the problem. He could have had a major problem.

Dr. John Christopher recommending using Plantain to draw toxin out when one has stepped on a nail. He mixed the crushed or dried leaves with Olive Oil and applied it to the bottom of the foot. As the Oil dried or was absorbed, a fresh poultice of Plantain would be applied until the redness was gone.

Using this same factor, Sister Ann Marie contacted me about a foot problem. She has diabetes and one of her legs was already taken off a few years ago but she is fighting to keep the second one. I went to visit her and her foot was dark red and disfigured to the point of looking like a sweet potato. It was strange that the red and swelling didn't go up her leg but stayed only on the foot. She wanted very much to keep this leg. On the heal of this foot was an ulcerated sore, so my first suggestion was to apply Plantain salve to that area. I suggested that she could do this every night and because it would weep, she would have to make sure she had material that would absorb the liquid draining out. During the daytime, I suggested that she get the circulation going in that foot and the way she was going to do it was to alternate between hot and cold water baths in the day time.

I didn't get back to see her for a month but when I did, the ulcerated sore was puckered white scar tissue and the foot was its normal shape and color. She told me that the doctor that checks on her was amazed and told her to keep doing whatever it was that she was doing as it looked great.

The Christopher Herb Company makes an ointment that contains Plantain, called Black Ointment. I have used it on boils and staph infections to "draw them up" for identification. My sister showed me something on her hand and wanted to know what it was. I applied the Black Ointment and in three days I could tell her what it was and we could treat it.

Usually it takes about three days of applying the Black Ointment to bring the boil to the breaking point. After it has opened one must allow the "anger" to weep by continuing to draw it out with the ointment. When this is done, it is time for healing and the drawing ointment is replaced with a healing ointment.

Ointments can be made by putting plant material into some Olive Oil and simmering it for a while, then straining the plant material out. In some cases the plant material can be left in the oil and when cooled, used for the purpose it was intended.

When making a salve, one follows the preceding instructions and after the plant material is removed from the oil, Beeswax is put in to firm up the remaining matter.

Plantain can be used in the winter by drying it and putting the dried material into clean glass jars with labels. Dried Plant works as well as the fresh plant. Historically it was used to reduce swelling and it reduces the heat along with the pain of inflammation.

Having checked Dr. Duke's Database, I find that this plant contains almost 80 constituents to keep it in balance; it has something for everything from Anticancer elements to some that are sedative and some that dilate the veins.

When we use whole plants our bodies have been giving choices for healing.

Purslane

Portulaca oleracea

Last week I visited the Sear's gardening center. Their idea of gardening is similar to present day medical treatments. Kill and remove whatever is a bother and add chemicals to assist the rest to stay healthy.

I looked at the Ortho list of pest-plants and noted that over half were my very best friends. So I picked one on the list to tell you about.

Purslane is a weed that most people pull out of their gardens and throw away. She is small and likes to live in tilled soil. You find her around your roses or under your tomato plants. She lies close to the ground and sends her "branches" horizontal to the ground in all directions from the central root. The tiny yellow flowers sit in a rosette of leaves.

The parts that make her stand out from all the other weeds are her leaves. They are a lot like the leaves of a Jade plant or a very small oval aloe leaf. It is just this difference from the other weeds that endears her to an herbalist, for held within these leaves is Omega-3 fatty acid.

Omega-3 fatty acids are essential for every cell in the body. They have even been thought to inhibit breast and other forms of cancers.

One of my friends had a loss of skin pigment and wanted to know if there was an herbal combination that might be helpful. I consulted The School of Natural Healing and was reminded of Purslane with is fatty acids. It was suggested to use some of the herbs that are stimulants to get the nutrition to the cells that most needed these fatty acids. So I suggested herbs like Cayenne, Ginger, and Peppermint to get things moving.

The juice of Purslane has been used like Aloe for burns, and in combination with rose oil it has been used in the mouth for sores and loose teeth.

Purslane is also used for cardiac weakness. In some places it is even prescribed for this purpose.

The seeds are sometimes used for difficult breathing. I have found seeds to be very powerful foods. They contain all of the wonderful things that the plant contains and are ready to be sent into the next generation.

Because it is so rich in vitamins and minerals, Mrs. Grieves mentioned "that 2 to 3 ounces of Purslane a day was sufficient for a man even while undergoing great fatigue." I find this amazing and yet I have seen plants do such wonderful things in a short period of time that my surprise should be lost.

As a fresh cut herb in a salad, it adds a cooling effect to any meal. The older shoots can be put into stews and soups; they can even be pickled with salt and vinegar to have in the winter time.

In Europe this plant is cultivated for just this purpose. When used with Sorrel in equal parts, the French make a wonderful soup called "bonne femme"

Just think of all this nutrition that we have been throwing out or into our compost piles all these years. Herbs have so much to offer us in the way of healing and as we have just learned, as food. Why would we "Ortho" them?

Queen Anne's Lace

Daucus carota

In the winter's snow one sees sentinels sticking up, skeletons of the past summer and one of them is Queen Anne's Lace. This is a member of the carrot family; no this is the carrot family. The carrots that we now eat have all been bred from this lovely lady.

My neighbors asked me what this lacy flower was that had popped up in their garden. I pull it out and ask them to smell the root and tell me. A carrot smells like a carrot by any name.

This carrot is editable but it has a very bitter taste compared to the ones that we buy in the store. I guess you could call this a survival food.

This plant will grow up to five feet tall in the fields and roadsides. One of the things that my students are interested in is calcium and other minerals so we talk about how plants take minerals into themselves from the earth. When they are no longer living, this is when we find these plants of the past with their minerals left behind. It is the same with any plant, maple furniture is made from wood and the wood is what the plant left behind, the minerals that they used when they were alive. When one eats a plant, we are talking in minerals that have been used by that plant and these minerals are cell sized.

I recently saw an ad for calcium from Oyster shells. Have these been ground up to cell size and will your cells be able to use them? Probably not because they won't be combined with all the trace minerals that would be found in plants that are needed to make calcium usable, that is without choking your cells. The body knows that it needs these minerals so it sometimes parks them until the body can figure out how to get the particles made smaller. (It takes acid to break down minerals.) It parks the minerals in the joints and places like along the artery walls as in Atherosclerotic (Artery Plaque) or arteriosclerosis (Hardening of the arteries).

The lacy flower head is what I find interesting. I took my granddaughter out to see the weeds in my yard (And there is always a Queen Anne's Lace growing); I showed her these flowers. In this umbrella form made up of tiny flowers, at the very center is one small deep-purple floret. It is the signature of this plant, all the lace and in the middle is a drop of blood? When the flower is done, the spokes of this umbrella will start to close into a cup-shape or a bird's nest. They are beautiful in any way that you find them. I like using these in dried flower arrangements as they have a very up-right look to them.

There is another plant that looks a lot like Queen Anne's Lace but is poisonous. The difference is that Water Hemlock has a smooth stem with purple blotches on it. So if one is going to use a plant like this for food or medicine, remember that Queen Anne's Lace has coarse hairs on her all green stems. This is very important to remember as the other one is *poisonous*.

Next summer, pull one of the hairy green stems up and smell the root. It has a pungent carrot smell but is much smaller and more slender than our domestic carrot. According to Mrs. Grieves, "it has an acid disagreeable taste" and that puts it into the medicinal category. Now let's find out what it can do. Dr. Duke says that "Science confirms its bactericidal, diuretic, hypotensive, and worm-expelling properties." The seeds of these small florets are "Very useful in flatulence, windy colic, hiccough, dysentery, chronic coughs, etc."

So here is a beautiful, healing weed. Enjoy her everywhere you see her.

Red Clover

Trifolium pratense

One of the first introductions that I had to herbs was with Red Clover. These little plants have been around all my life. It is so surprising to find out just how powerful these soft red flowers are.

I first read about Red Clover while reading BACK TO EDEN by Jethro Kloss. Did you know that Kloss grew up in Manitowoc, Wisconsin? He talked about being sent by his parents to gather the blossoms for their "postmaster, who had a serious cancer. He (The postmaster) lived to be a rather old man, without an operation." I think that is when I decided that herbs could do some very important things. Herbs are so wonderful!

Kloss suggests that it is excellent for cancer in any part of the body. He even has a formula that is: 1 ounce Red Clover blossoms, 1 ounce Burdock seed, 2 ounces Wild Oregon Grape root, and 1/2 ounce Bloodroot root. He suggests mixing them in one pint of hot water and one pint of hot apple cider. Cover and let stand for a couple of hours, and then use 4 ounces, four times a day.

With throat cancer, he suggests gargling with this formula four or five times a day and swallowing some of the tea.

Wherever the cancer is located on the body, that part should be bathed five to six times a day with this formula.

I remember my mentor, Hanna Kroeger mentioning that four ounces of anything goes right into the blood stream. She said that more of anything didn't.

That wasn't the only reference that I found connecting cancer to Red Clover. The "Flower tea is drunk daily for breast cancer, and the whole plant is included in experimental treatments for diverse cancers," according to Lesley Bremness in the EYEWITNESS HANDBOOK – HERBS.

Research shows that there are compounds in Red Clover that inhibit some laboratory tumors. Scientists are trying to catch up with herbalist and prove things that are already so.

Kloss even suggested that Red Clover is splendid for handling Syphilis.

Red Clover is one of the great blood cleansers of the herbal kingdom. As a blood cleanser it doesn't screen the blood but cleans the cells that are loaded with toxins and gives them nourishment.

There has been some research that Red Clover is helpful for Thrombosis as an Anticoagulant.

Red Clover is good for Whooping Cough and Bronchial problems along with Arthritis and skin complaints.

When we think of a clear, hot tea doing all the things that have been mentioned here, it is hard to imagine, but herbal teas have been doing this for hundreds of years with amazing results. Why do we think that only "hard on the body" heavy radiation or chemicals will eliminate cancers?

Red Clover is so identifiable. The three oval leaflets have a chevron of light green on them. The red flower petals on the composite heads can be pulled off one at a time or in a group. The base of the petals are sweet. The bees know just what they are doing when they head for Red Clover.

Did you know that white Clover has been made into feed for animals and that the flowers were once made into bread? Herbs are food.

Our yard is full of white clover and I so enjoy sitting on the lawn at night in the summer with the white flower heads picking up any light around. This makes the yard look like it has stars all over it.

Clover puts nitrogen into the soil so having it in my yard is an added bonus.

Red Raspberry

Rubus strigosus

This plant is related to roses.

Most herbalist use the leaves in tea form due to their nutritive properties. This tea is a great agent for cleansing the mucus membranes in the G.I. tract, leaving the tissues toned. It is great for cleaning up canker conditions.

Dr. Christopher recommends distilled water with Red Raspberry leaf tea for three days to clean the system when one has a cold sore. He also recommends this tea to wash foreign particles out of the eye. In the process it will act as an astringent and heal the irritated surface.

The tea is so gentle that it can be used for children's complaints of stomachaches. Taken regularly will quiet premature pains in pregnancy and will produce a safe, speedy and easy delivery.

When nursing a baby for a long time and the baby doesn't seem to be satisfied, Christopher recommends that Mom drinking Red Raspberry leaf tea along with Marshmallow Root to enrich the contents of the milk.

As teenagers grow up, they are blamed for not being cooperative. Their bodies are craving vitamins and minerals that are not found in a teen's diet. They are eating fast foods, sweet and excessive meats. Their bodies react with acne, boils and irritability. Girls have more difficult periods. Boys have to deal with an unhealthy sex drive. A cup of Red Raspberry leaf tea will assist in supplying natural hormone materials to their bodies, thus allowing them to attain a balance.

When harvesting Red Raspberry leaves, the best time is before noon but after the morning dew is gone. The best seasons are Spring and Summer when the berries are not on the plant. Never strip a plant of all its leaves as these are where they process their food. Take a few from each plant.

To dry these leaves, one might lay them out in a shady but airy place and cover with cheese cloth to keep the bugs out. Another way is to place them into a large paper bag and close the top. Label the bag, and then shake this up daily while turning the bag onto a different side daily. The bottom will become moist and wick the moisture out of the leaves without harboring parasites.

When your leaves are completely dry, put them into a glass jar and label your jar. Now when you are making tea, you can use a tablespoon in a cup of hot water. This tea has been use for such things as thrush, scurvy, morning sickness, gout, flu, acid indigestion, skin ulcers, fevers, vomiting, and wounds.

Let's talk about the berries of this plant. The fruit contains acids along with minerals and fruit sugars. The coloring matter contains flavonoids which are found in many fruits with dark coloring in them. (This is similar to the purple found in grape skins.) This property is what makes these fruits so good for the heart. The coloring matter has also been used for dying purposes.

According to what I have read, "Raspberry contains three times as much cellulose and less ash than strawberries" (Christopher) This ash consists of calcium, magnesium, potassium, phosphorus, sulfur and iron.

A homemade wine can be easily made from the raspberries. It is said to be anti-scrofulous, which means that it will help the lymphatic system.

I have saved the best for last. Under the direction of Dr. Daniel Nixon; Dr. Dave Gangemi of Hollings Cancer Center in Charleston, South Carolina put out some information on a study that he and a colleague completed. He said that his study showed that the Elliagic Acid in Red Raspberry seeds will cause (G-arrest) stop breast cancer in 48 hours (Inhibiting and stopping mitosis-cancer cell division) and reverse it in 72 hours. This is presently being checked out for pancreas, esophageal, skin, colon and prostate cancer cells. I sent for his information on this study and he returned the paperwork to me.

That should have been the end of that but a research doctor in the State of Washington didn't believe this so he did his own independent study and got the same results. A female research doctor from Loyola in Illinois decided to see if this could be so. She got the same results as the other two did.

Dr. Susan Thorpe-Vargas states, "Multiple studies have discovered that Phytonutrients found in raspberries can protect us from cancer and can even shrink some types of cancer tumors." She goes on to say, "Recent work(2001), published by Dr. Gary Stoner at Ohio State University, showed that components in the seeds and berry, but particularly ellegitannins, inhibited the initation and promotion/progression stages of esophageal cancer." "In addition, edible berries, including raspberries also inhibit angiogenesis. This is a term used to describe the development of blood vessels needed for tumor growth." This from SCIENTIFIC MEDICAL DEVICES, Inc. Cumming, GA.

My questions are: if these research doctors got this kind of results independently, why are we still funding breast cancer research?

Why are we still removing breasts?

Why aren't doctors allowed to use any of this information?

When is the American Medical Association, the American Cancer Association and all the rest going to wake up and allow us to use information found with the research monies that all those "Pink" ribbons are for? Are only the Cancer Centers of America allowed to use what works?

This acid is found in Raspberries, Strawberries and Walnuts. Be sure to chew/bite the seeds.

Roses

Rose canina

Everything is coming up roses and why not? It is the end of the season and time to harvest rosehips. The last of the flower petals have fallen and the base of the rose flower has expanded to give us a pod with seeds in it.

Today I cut the hips off my rose bushes to dry and save them for January and February when I will have a wonderful rosehip tea, loaded with 16 different constituents according to Dr. James Duke's data base. Along with all the Vitamin A, D, E and C that they contain, I found them to be AntiAlzheimer, Antibacterial, Anticataract, AntiCrohn's, Antidiabetic and Antioxident. The data base also mentioned that rosehips were heavy into cancer prevention and also Antiviral. As an added bonus, they contain iron for women who are always looking for a little extra from time to time.

Now what to do with these little round things, I slice the berry on one side so that it exposes the seeds. (By the way these seeds can be grown in your hot house to make new plants.) Next I put the pods on a cookie sheet and into my oven that is set on warm. I like to put a wooden spoon in the door of the oven to keep it opened a crack which allows the humidity to escape. I check them every so often to make sure that they are drying. The seeds will come out very easily as the pod dries with just a slight scraping. When they are dry, I place the pod skins in a glass jar and label it so that I have my vitamins ready for the winter.

In the winter, I can take a tablespoonful of these dried pods out, then put them in a small kettle of water. I simmer them for about 10 minutes and relive my roses of the summer in the form of a wonderful tart tea. For those of you who like it sweeter, you might add a couple Stevia or Peppermint leaves to this tea.

These dried pods can be added to soups and stews in the wintertime for the whole family to benefit. Think of all the colds and flu your family can avoid with all this natural stuff.

Roses are for any time of the year.

Rosemary

Rosemarinus Officinalis

Here is an interesting plant that I have used to help my mother. Mom had a stroke on the left side of her brain. Her right leg and her right arm were affected with her right hand forming a ball and curl into her chest. I didn't really understand the body effects but I wanted to help Mom.

I remembered reading in Mrs. Grieve's book A MODERN HERBAL about Dandelion or Rosemary helping one of the royals in Europe that also had a stroke, a few hundred years ago. So it was back to the books for me. I found it! It seems that fresh Rosemary was cut and put into "Spirits of wine, this was allowed to stand for four days and then distilled." According to Mrs. Grieve this formula was "dated 1235, said to be in the handwriting of Elizabeth, Queen of Hungary." It was to be taken in small amounts like a tonic. (Tonics are taken once a day in a capsule or as a tablespoonful. "Tonics are herbs that stimulate nutrition and permanently increase systemal tone, energy, vigor, and strength," according to Dr. John Christopher.)

After finding this again, I decided to try it. I make dandelion wine in accordance with an old family recipe given to me by my Dad's cousin. Having a few bottles of this homemade wine, I cut tops off my Rosemary and dropped them into the wine to allow the wine to pull all of the active ingredients into it. Then we started to administer this to Mom. Within a few days we noticed that her arm had relaxed into her lap and her hand wasn't tightly curled. She seemed more at ease and not so agitated. She was unable to talk to us at that time so I didn't know how it was making her feel.

My boss mentioned that she had a client only in her 20s that had recently had a stroke too. She asked me to make this formula for her client. I did and made a disclaimer for her client to sign. Not sure if it would have held up in court but I needed to protect myself in case of a problem.

I didn't hear anything about this client so I asked my boss. She didn't know how it had worked either but gave me her phone number. The client lived with her parents so I got to talk to her Mother. I was told that the client was sleeping, so I mentioned that I had created the herbal tonic and wanted to know how it was working. The Mother was raving about it. She said that before the tonic, this girl only slept about two hours at a time as she was in so much discomfort. When the tonic started to work and the muscles relaxes, she was able to sleep for long periods of time. The Dandelion and Rosemary had released the torqued muscles.

Because Rosemary is so good at stimulating circulation it can be used for headaches, nervous diseases. I even read where it will help with kidney problems.

Dr. Duke in his book THE GREEN PHARMACY talks about it being used for Alzheimer's due to its antioxidant properties. He even mentions that it is sometimes called the "Herb of remembrance."

Duke mentions that Rosemary has properties that can be used to preserve foods without refrigeration. This is an interesting idea. We usually associate Salt with this ability. In the old west they would dry or salt meats to keep them from becoming un-useable, now we know that Rosemary has this capability also.

Rosemary has such a wonderful clean smell to it, almost a Pine smell, if you will. I decided to look in Dr. Duke's wonderful Database and see what is creating this wonderful smell. I found that 23 different constituents in this one herb, accounts for this smell. He labels them with the word, "perfumery".

Last week I decided to put Rosemary simmered in Olive oil on my hair, mainly to get the tangles out and found that it added a wonderful smell. For reasons unknown to me or anyone, I have not had my hair cut for three years so it tends to get tangled up and the tangles were easy to undo with this combination. I guess it might also help my brain and stimulate the circulation in the scalp with this combination, not a bad side effect.

While I was in Duke's Data base, I wanted to see what this plant is capable of doing. I found so many things that were Anticancerous, Antibacterial, Antiinflammatory. I bumped into Antiviral many times and Antisalmonella was there along with Antilymphomic and Antirhinoviral. Even AntiSyndrome-X was in there, a precursor of Diabetes.

I can truly understand why this is such a wonderful herb and in my area, I can have it in a pot in my house all winter long. So what am I going to do with this herb? After reading all the things that this wonderful lady can do, I think that every time I water her or clean around her, I will ask her permission for me to take one of her pungent leaves. Chewing on this will give my body a good feeling because not only am I able to ingest all of the constituents in this plant but I have been given a gift from this plant.

Sassafras

Sassafras officinale

Every spring I start out my spring house cleaning with me. I put a tablespoonful of Sassafras root into a kettle along with distilled water and simmer it for a while. As this reddish-brown root simmers, the volatile oils permeate my house. When it has simmer for a while (So what is a while, maybe half an hour to a whole hour.) I allow it to cool enough for me to sip on it. Dr. Christopher mentioned that while it is hot it will act as a diaphoretic. Sometimes that is needed in a spring house cleaning to get all the skin pores cleaned out.

Everything I have read about this herb talks about using it to mask disagreeable and bitter tastes of other herbs by combining it with them. I have to tell you that of itself, it is not a wonderful tasting herb. It has the smell and taste of varnish. I do a lot of woodworking and I know what varnish smells like, have never tasted it but if it has a taste, that is what it would taste like. (Although coffee smells great but doesn't have that great taste.)

Sassafras does more than just taste strangely. It goes to work to help the body in many ways. According to Dr. John R. Christopher, It is "an antidote for poisoning by acid or alkaline corrosives." He also mentioned that it kills protozoa, a single celled parasite that we can pick up from just about anywhere. Gardeners pick them up a lot.

It contains tannic acids, gums, albumen, starch, lignin, resin, wax, heavy and light volatile oils, camphorous matter and salts.

Dr. Christopher mentions all the things that it is capable of handling, such as: skin diseases, rheumatism, scrofula, impure blood, Syphilis, poison-ivy, poison- oak, tobacco poisoning, colds, amenorrhea, ophthalmia (Inflamed eyes), spasms, pain in the heart region, colic, flatulence, problems of the kidneys, bladder, chest & throat, and as a tonic after childbirth.

Dr. C. says that "it is a blood purifier. The safrole is a trace mineral extremely important and will clean the heart, arteries, veins and cut cholesterol while giving elasticity to the veins. It is to be used ONLY IN ITS WHOLESOME STATE of Sassafras Bark Tea. The safrole should *never* be used alone but as a whole plant. It is very good in a tea for edema as it steps up the circulation and makes the heart sound."

According to Jethro Kloss author of BACK TO EDEN, the oil of Sassafras is excellent for toothaches and is a great external wash for varicose ulcers. He also recommended it as a tonic for stomach and bowels.

Looks like I could be using this many times a year instead of just in the spring.

Let's jump back to the word WHOLESOME. A lot of chemicals are found in "health food stores" but they are not the whole herb, they are just one of the chemicals that someone thought was most active. When we pull things apart, we start to get side effects but when we use the whole herb, all of the constituents that comprise this plant work together to help us heal without side effects.

Everyone that wrote about this herb had warnings about it. Dr. C. says, "Do not use over 6 weeks at a time, change to another like it, maybe Morman Tea or Red Clover Tea." Kloss on the other hand mentions that it should be taken for no more than a week and he recommends it being taken as a tincture in water.

Now we get to have a look at the other side of this. There was a Lilly Distinguished Professor of Pharmacognosis at Purdue University. I have Dr. Varro E. Tyler's book HERBS OF CHOICE and I always check to see what he has to say coming from the Pharmaceutical perspective. Sometimes I believe that he is against all herbs but let's see what he had to say about Sassafras. "Sassafras root contains 5 to 9 % safrole shown to be a carcinogenic in rats and mice." He mentions that in 1976 the FDA prohibited its sale. He said that it is "Not safe" and compared it to Comfrey,

Coltsfoot, Borage and Mistletoe. (I also write about some of these. One of my favorites is Comfrey.) He mentioned that "Sarsaparilla and Sassafras are ineffective and dangerous."

You don't think that they tested one of the chemicals on rats, namely Safrole and found that alone it is dangerous? Again I want to stress only using *WHOLE* plants and herbs to give the body what it needs to repair itself.

I checked Nova Scotia Museum's Poison Plant Database and could not find Sassafras listed.

I decided to check Dr. James A. Duke's Database on this and found 33 different components in the roots of Sassafras. He had many more in the leaves and stems of this plant but because I use only the roots, that is what I am writing about. With all the good stuff that these 33 things do such as being; Antibacterial, Antiinflammatory, Antioxidant, (I even found Antistreptococcic), Antisalmonella, Antiviral, cancerpreventive, Candidicide, Cardioprotective and as a Vasodilator;

(Some heavy stuff.) I did find four things that would make this an herb not to take while pregnant.

We have heard from all the "good guys" and as you can see, even they don't recommend anyone staying on Sassafras for a long period of time. I try to put both sides in my writings and think it is time to simmer some Sassafras tea for me to sip on today.

Before I finish this writing, I remembered that I had heard of Sassafras as being a blood thinner but haven't been able to confirm this as of yet. The most that I can find out is that in the spring, this plant puts out chemicals that thin the blood but in the fall its chemicals tend to thicken the blood. When buying Sassafras at a health food store, are you getting spring root or fall root?

Always use your good judgment. If you have a health care provider that suggests something, do the research and find out all you can about whatever they have suggested. We have become a society that wants someone else to be responsible for us and our health. We need to take back that power and help ourselves. I write these articles to give more information so that we can make good decisions for our health and the health of our families.

Shepherd's Purse

Capsella Bursa

One year I had an interesting weed growing in my garden. I decided to see who it was. I allowed it to continue to grow and when it was 18 inches high, it flowered. I still didn't know who he was. Then he had seeds and I knew. Who could mistake the seed pods of Shepherd's Purse? Their leaves look like wild lettuce but the seed pods dangle along the branches and are flat with heart-shapes. They are a member of the mustard family and are found in waste lands all over.

My thought was to find out what part of this plant was used medicinally and harvest just that part. I thought I would be harvesting the seed pods or maybe the roots, but I was surprised to learn that the "herb" is what one uses. This means that the whole plant is used. The stalk, leaves, roots and seeds.

Alma Hutchins, talks about this plant in her book, INDIAN HERBALOGY OF NORTH AMERICA. The first thing that I learned from her was that the American Indians used this plant for food. They ate the leaves raw or cooked and the seed pods were collected and roasted. Sometimes they added them to another meal, perhaps ground up acorns and made a type of bread.

Out of the 60 constituents that I found in this plant, some of them have the ability to stop bleeding by coagulating blood. Dr. Mowrey talked about it lowering blood pressure in his book THE SCIENTIFIC VALIDATION OF HERBAL MEDICINE. Dr. Mowrey suggested using the fresh or dried whole plant as a tea.

According to Mrs. Grieves book, A MODERN HERBAL, in "The Great War", when medicine ran out, a tea and poultice of Shepherd's Purse was used on the soldiers. They even made an ointment of it "especially for head wounds."

Ointments are made by heating vegetable oil (Extra Virgin Olive Oil) and simmering it with the herb in. After it has simmer for about 20 to 30 minutes, strain the herb out of the oil and return the oil to the pot. While still on low heat, add beeswax until a spoonful of this mixture can be tested in a cool place. (Refrigerate for 3 minutes.) The consistency will be just as it will be when it has cooled naturally. If it is too hard, add a little more oil. If it is too runny, add more wax.

Because of its ability to stop bleeding, it will check hemorrhoids. This can be done by putting the juice of Shepherd's Purse on cotton and inserting it or by making a little of the ointment with more wax and harden it into a suppository.

Dr. James Duke's database talks about all of its abilities and they surprised me. I would just like to mention a few of the things that this plant can do. In the Database I ran into its Anticancer ability many times. I found cardio protection in there and Antiinflammatory along with Antibacterial properties. Antioxident was there as was Antidiabetic but one thing that really surprised me was pituitary-stimulant. I might, in the future go back into the database to find out what of the 60 properties had this particular ability but as everyone knows, I am big on whole herbs so I guess that is what is really important. The next time one of these grows in my gardens, I will nibble on one of its leaves.

In the folk medicine department I found that it had been used for stomach ulcers, kidney and bladder problems (especially when bleeding is involved), and lung problems such as Tuberculosis, also as a tincture for typhoid fever.

Our weeds are so valuable. Enjoy learning about them and making medicine with them.

Slippery Elm

Ulmus Fulva

Here is another not so little herb, Slippery Elm bark. I have put this one on my "Big Guns" list because of all the wonderful things it is capable of doing.

Let's start with its ability to rebuild body parts. Dr. John R. Christopher, of Utah mentioned that Slippery Elm has the ability to rebuild the body. He went on to talk about how a poultice of Slippery Elm bark powder could be applies to hips or knees to rebuild these parts. What Slippery Elm does is supply all the building blocks to that area. He suggested keeping this poultice moist and allowing the body to absorb it. When it is absorbed it was suggested to reapply it. He mentioned that one would never need to take any of the old poultice off as the body was using this to rebuild the area where it was being applied. I find that just amazing.

The American Natives used tree bark in a similar manner. They would cut a strip of bark off the tree and tie it to an injured area then just go on with their lives. The inner bark of a tree is where the tree's blood is; so in putting this next to an injury, one is giving the body the benefit of a blood transfusion, so to speak from the tree. David Christopher, director of the School of Natural Healing mentioned that the difference between plant blood and human blood is only one thing. Sorry but at this point in my life, I don't remember what it was, iron, potassium or what.

Slippery Elm bark powder has the nutritional value equivalent to oatmeal. It can be used to support life at an early age. When a baby is not eating or not gaining weight properly, Slippery Elm gruel can be given to it by making a very runny gruel. In the same manner, when an elderly person is not able to assimilate their food, Slippery Elm gruel can be eaten. The properties are able to rebuild the cells of the body. Slippery Elm bark powder does not like to combine with water easily so one has to create gruel by adding one drop of water at a time to a pile of Slippery Elm powder. Rolling this drop around until it has collected some of the powder and then adding another drop until you have collected all of the powder. Now, one can make it into anything that is needed by adding more water if necessary.

Slippery Elm powder can be made into suppositories to heal the vaginal area or to heal hemorrhoids. While checking Dr. Duke's database, I found one constituent in this herb that was "Antivaginitic". (Dr. Duke's word.) I also found a lot of Anticancer constituents. This herb is on my "big Guns" list for a lot of reasons.

A few years ago a lady called me. She was very upset because she had burned her arm while burning off the land behind her house. Her first thought (and we are trained to think this way) was to go to the doctor. He put a chemical healer on the burn and told her to come back in 10 days. She followed his advice and went back. She had just gotten back from her doctor's visit this second time when she called me. Well, she had taken time to talk to a nurse who was a student of mine and the nurse suggested that she call me. She told me that at the doctor's office, they did a debridement. "Surgical removing of dead or contaminated tissue and foreign matter from a wound" from the Heritage College Dictionary – Third Edition. They had removed the old scabs that had formed on top of the burned area. This is standard practice for handling burns by the medical field. When the body is in the process of healing a wound, it forms a scab. This is God's way of protecting this injured area from contaminates. Why would the medical profession know better than GOD?

I mentioned that she might want to start the healing with Slippery Elm on the raw flesh. Then I mentioned the Health Food Store in her area where she would be able to get the Slippery Elm. I also mentioned that it needed to be kept moist and she could call me anytime. She called back later that day and asked what to do next. Thinking that she had used Slippery Elm Powder, I suggested that she reapply it to the affected area. It seems that the Health Food

Store sold her bark hunks as they told her that the powder would not mix with water.

Now she had to soak the arm and allow the bark to come out of the "trying to heal already" flesh and I gave her instructions on how to get to my house. When she arrived, we made a paste of Slippery Elm Powder and spread it on the raw flesh, covered this with damp cotton and plastic to keep it moist. I gave her a small jar of Slippery Elm Powder to take home until she could get some of her own.

I told her that when this scabs over again, we will treat the area with something else.

I got a call from a lady from Plymouth. She told me that a friend had told her to call me to get help for her son. It seems that this four year old had fallen into a pile of burning leaves and had burned his lower legs. She wanted to know if I would be willing to help him. I asked her where he was and she mentioned that he was in the hospital. I told her that I would love to help but that I am not allowed to do anything in hospitals. She mentioned that it was killing her and her husband as they hugged each other while the staff debrides their son's legs every other day and he is screaming even while under morphine. I also explained that if they were to take their son out of the hospital to give him a different kind of care, the social system would take the child away from them as the only system of medical care that is recognized at the present time is from Doctors and hospitals. It was all that I could give her at this time.

Slippery Elm rebuilds flesh but it contains constituents that have the following properties; Candidicide, Anticancer, Antibacterial, Antiaging, Pesticide and many more.

Why is "Pesticide" important? Because we are constantly confronted with parasites in our water, our food and our environment. It is wonderful that some of our foods have the ability to eliminate some of these parasites and yes, herbs are foods. Actually, I believe that they make the environment in our bodies less attractive to the life cycle of parasites. Many plants have this ability but most of the plants that we eat are eaten cooked, so taking an herbal tea or capsule is most helpful from time to time.

Herbs are food so let your medicine be your food and your food be your medicine.

Sᴛ. John'sᴡoʀᴛ
ᕼypᴇʀicum pᴇʀꜰoʀᴀᴛum

In this chapter I wish to share some information on St. John'swort. It isn't a native in the Americas; like my ancestors, it came from Europe. It is my feeling that if something is important enough to bring with you when you move to another place, there must be something special about it, and there is.

It was used as a nervine to assist in healing injured nerves, even sciatica. It is very helpful when in excessive pain. What we have been taught is that it is just used for depression.

In the last few years St. John'swort has gotten a bad name for itself but it wasn't the plant's fault. As an Antidepressant in popular use, it was standardized for its hypericin.

When pharmacists standardized this plant, they try to find out what of the 60+ constituents is helpful for...let's say depression. They came up with hypericin and decide to make sure that the product they are selling you is loaded with this one compound. Now that sounds good except this is now a chemical composition and not an herbal product. They did this same thing with aspirin/ the salicylic acid from plants. Man always thinks they can do a better job. In an herbal product all the compounds are in balance with each other so that none will create "side effect" for the most part. The St. John'swort that has been sold in the last few years is made in a chemical factory and is sold under the name of St. John'swort. It is a drug and is harmful to the body.

We have a wonderful plant that has small green leaves and grows wild. In July it bursts into flower with wonderful small yellow flowers. It is so wonderful that the American Indian would dry it and grind it up like corn meal to make food. They also knew about its healing effects on the nerves. One book that I read even mentioned that a lot of early cooks would put some of this dried plant into their homemade bread and found that the bread was even better that way. St. John'swort was found to be so mild that it could be used for people of all ages from small children to adults. With children it has been said to help with bed wetting, with adults it has been credited with cleaning up bronchial problems. A tea of St. John'swort can be used to heal the mouth and teeth area.

I decided to head into Dr. James Duke's Phytochemical and Ethnobotanical Databases for some answers as to just what wonderful things this plant is capable of helping me with. I decided to pick out only the constituents where more than one of the 60+ did the same things. Here is what St. John'swort is able to do: it is an AntiAlzheimeran, Antibacterial, Anticataract, Antidementia, Antidiabetic, Antiflu, Antiinflammatory, Antioxident, Antispasmodic, Antiulcer, Antiviral , and fungicide. Along with those talents, it is a cancer preventive, is capillariprotective, also a pesticide and a Vasodilator. Hey, if only three of these compounds have the ability to keep me from having cataracts, I think it is wonderful.

I found that many of the compounds in this herb are sedative and a few are photosensitizers. I mention this last one because I have read about how eating or using this product will affect one's skin regarding the sun. The funny thing is that I also found compounds that act as sunscreens built right into the same plant. It is amazing how these plants were designed without the help of man to balance themselves out?

St John'swort has been called many names: Goatweed, Hypericum, Klamath weed, and St John'swort. In some places, predators have been imported to get rid of it because some animals have developed skin problems after eating a lot of it. The same report that gave me this information said that humans are not sensitive in this way.

I should mention that if you are taking some form of drug, you might not want to add St. John'swort to your list but that is a given. Why would you be mixing drugs with herbal remedies?

I see a product that is helpful in many ways in my life and it will remain in my medicine chest as a tincture to be used as needed for any of the above. Sometime we need to look at the big picture before we make a judgment about things. It is also a good thing to learn to make your own medicine, that way you know just what is in the product.

Stevia

Stevia rebaudiana

Tonight a plant was screaming at me. They tend to do that when I'm too busy to give them the attention that they want.

This little plant is a real sweetie and I mean that literally. Her name is Stevia and tonight she was trying to get my attention to show me some tiny white flowers. No wonder she wanted water. She isn't hard to grow in a pot sitting on a windowsill most of the time and she gives me a leaf or two all the time.

Stevia has a substance called Stevioside in it that is said to be as much as 250 times as sweet as sucrose and 50 times sweeter than sugar. Tests show that the Stevioside is heat stable, pH stable and non-fermentable. (Looks like I will have to use regular sugar for making my wines.)

There are about 250 plants in this genus of the sunflower family. They are found growing all over South America, Central America and in the southern part of North America.

All studies repeat that she is safe for Diabetics to use as she contains _no_ sugar. She will not interfere with anyone dealing with Candida either.

In the past I have contacted the American Diabetes Association and asked why they recommend aspartame for Diabetics and their response came in a letter. They said basically, "There continues to be unsubstantiated claims that the non-nutritive sweetener aspartame (Brand name NutraSweet) poses health risks to people with Diabetes."

Most countries recognize this sweetener, in Japan Stevia makes up 40% of their sweetener market.

The United States has restricted it to being labeled as a dietary supplement but not a food additive. Both Coca-Cola and PepsiCo are producing a commercial product and hope to be able to get the "Food Additive" label approved by the government. As of December 2008, the FDA has lifted the ban on Stevia under pressure from companies like Coca Cola and Pepsi. This is a real win for those of us who will not use anything with aspartame. I have even seen an ad for Stevia calling the product Truvia. Isn't it interesting what big business can do?

Dr. Duke's Database showed me things that are contained in this plant and are known to be Cardioprotective and Cancer-preventive along with a whole lot more.

When I give a person a leaf to taste, I always take one myself so that they know it is safe to eat. Most people are surprised by the taste. First comes the sweet taste and then it is balanced out. Nature never over does what is needed.

Try two Stevia leaves for dessert tonight or plan to adopt a member of her family.

Stinging Nettle

Urtica dioica

Let me tell you about a most maligned friend of mine called Stinging Nettle.

Here we have a 3 to 6 foot plant with nothing about it to show its value. It has no big pretty flowers; instead the flowers are tiny and green. It has no unusual leaves to give it a "must save" value. So to defend itself, it has stiff, stinging hairs on the outside of the leaves and on the stems. I had an herbalist call me to her house once because she told me that her Stinging Nettle wasn't stinging. And I found that they were very gentle plants. I had to work to get them to sting me. (Talking to plants is a subject for Part Two of this book.) What most people don't know is that it also contains an antidote to its stings and herein lies the treasure.

The spine of the leaf contains this antidote. While on an herbal walk in Utah, our instructor showed us how to eat fresh Nettle leaves. You pick the leaf by touching the spine on the back of the leaf. The leaf is then folded into itself, exposing the back of the leaf and breaking the leaf's spine. The secret is the very last part, breaking the spine. The juice of this spine counteracts the Nettle's poison or stings. In fact, this juice will counteract the poison of other plants as well.

It will act on Poison Ivy and Poison Oak. A friend of mine had large blisters all over one foot and up his leg. He told me it was Poison Ivy. I suggested that he try Stinging Nettle Tea on it. He called later that day and was very happy when the blisters started to go down as he applied the tea and within hours his leg was back to normal.

I have known of other people who have tried this and it took a couple of days. According to my teacher, Dr. Christopher, "Herbs work best on clean bodies." If the toxins get stopped on the way out of the body by a clogged-up lymph system or a malfunctioning liver or constipated bowels, they tend to be recycled in the body. Most of the time when the normal ways out are clogged-up, they try to get out though the skin and one gets a "new rash" in another place. The skin is the largest organ of the human body.

An old rhyme tells of another way to handle the sting of Nettle. "Nettle in, Dock out, Dock rubs Nettle out." They are talking about Burdock and Yellow Dock. There are other herbs that handle the sting of Nettle too such as Rosemary and Sage leaves.

An interesting thing about Nettle is that once you dry it or cook it, it no longer stings on contact, but the other properties that make this a wonderful medicinal plant will still be there. Some of the chemical constituents are: "Formic acid (in fresh plants), mucilage, iron phosphate, potassium phosphate, magnesium phosphate and potassium chloride." The potassium phosphate is the basic food for our brain and nervous system. The potassium chloride is nature's masterpiece solvent of fibrin. On reading about this last talent, I think of how many people complain of Fibromyalgia, which basically is old muscle and skin fibers have not dissolved and been flushed away like they are designed to be. Perhaps Nettle could be used for this too?

I have read where decomposing wounds and ulcers have healed after using Nettle as a daily wash.

With all of these wonderful organic minerals, according to Jack Ritchason in the LITTLE HERB ENCYCLOPEDIA, "it has the ability to alleviate allergic symptoms such as teary eyes and running nose, as it is Antiasthmatic." Ritchason also mentioned that it improves functions in most body organs.

In the past Nettle tea was used to cure dandruff and bring back one's natural hair color.

One of the things I learned about Nettle was that its leaves are rich in iron which helps the formation of hemoglobin in the blood. It has been used to purify and rebuild the blood.

I also found the Nettle contains organic aluminum that is needed by the brain. The brain knows that it needs this so it steals it from your soda cans and aluminum foil. What I understand is that aluminum helps to create the connections in the brain. Organic Aluminum along with most organic things have the ability to go back and forth across the blood/ brain barrier but in-organic can't and a build-up of Aluminum is what is thought to create Alzheimer's disease. Lately I have been reading where they think that by taking in Silicon; it will help to remove the excess Aluminum. Nettle also contains organic Silicon. Isn't it interesting that nature (God) knew how to do this in the first place?

My friend Debbie asked about growing Stinging Nettle. I grow Stinging Nettle. It doesn't seem to need much gardening. Mine grows to three and a half feet tall but I have seen it as tall as five feet. I have mine in the middle of a twelve by twelve foot raised box garden. It likes "nitrogen-rich soil, wastelands". My original plants came from Baraboo Wisconsin and were growing on Elephant dung piles, created by the Baraboo Circus.

I also have raspberries growing in the same box as the nettle. We have deer in the area and they like to eat the tops of the raspberry stalks. I notice that when they hit the nettle, they no longer continue to nibble the raspberries plants.

The idea of putting Nettle in the middle of my raspberries was so that I can continue to have them in my yard and anyone viewing my gardens will not get stung. If you have ever been stung you know that this is not a pleasant thing. According to Ritchason, "The Indians used Nettle as a counter-irritant when in pain, by striking the affected part with the branches." This would bring the blood to that area and allow the healing to begin.

Ritchason mentioned that it was very beneficial for pregnant women due to being rich in Vitamin K. Vitamin K guards against excessive bleeding. He also mentioned that Nettle improves kidney function and prevents hemorrhoids.

On the fun side, in Europe Nettle beer has been made by combining it with other herbs. This was used for gout and rheumatic pains but it mostly was enjoyed as a refreshing drink.

The name Nettle means "textile plant". Nettle has been harvested like flax to be made into cloth. During the war many European countries grew and harvested it. It was thought (according to Ritchason) to be, "inferior to silk but much superior to cotton for velvet and plush."

I like a cup of Nettle tea a couple times a week. I like to add a little licorice root to my tea to sweeten it but as you can see, Nettle needs to be given a place of honor in your herbal medicine chest.

Strawberries

Fragaria vesca

As a child, we would go for walks in the summer, picking and eating the wild Strawberries that grew by the road side.

We would see all kinds of wild plants but the Strawberries were our favorites. Sometimes we would take a container along and collect enough of them to take home so Mom could make Strawberry short cake.

Wild Strawberries have a very distinct flavor. They are very tangy, quite unlike the large ones that we buy in the store today. Wild Strawberries are small and red most of the way through.

I allow weeds in my gardens and every so often I find a wild Strawberry that has migrated to my yard. They make a good ground cover for the places that always need help. That brings me to why they are called Strawberries. One would think it is because straw is laid under the berries to keep them off the ground but that is not so. According to Mrs. Grieves (a noted herbalist), they had the name long before this custom. It seems the verb "to stew" was changed to straw; this was referring to "the tangle of vines with which Strawberries cover the ground."

Did you know that Strawberries are a great blood purifier and that Strawberry juice combats bacterial infections? According to Dr. Christopher in his Natural Healing Newsletter Vol. 5 #1,

Strawberries are recommended for sluggish liver, gout, rheumatism, constipation, high blood pressure, skin cancer and Syphilis. (And we just thought they tasted good.) He also said that if one pound of Strawberries is eaten in the morning with no other food until noon, pinworms would often disappear. He mentioned that eating some at the beginning of a meal would stimulate the appetite.

With some people, Strawberries clean their system faster than the liver can process the toxins that are being flushed out. When this happens the toxins head for the skin, one of the four ways to get things out of the body. (Liver, Lungs, Bowels/Kidneys and Skin.) This makes people think that they are allergic to Strawberries since they get a rash when they eat them. What happens is that the Strawberries are doing a heavy cleansing. I recommend that people who think they are allergic to Strawberries, clean the bowels and liver first so when the toxins are released they will exit the body in an easy-normal way. (Another reason for an allergy to foods might be the chemicals that the farmer put on the plants to get a good harvest.)

Strawberries are high in iron and the leaf tea is used as a wash for skin problems such as eczema. Fresh berries can be rubbed over blackheads to assist the healing.

Another thing that is nice about Strawberries is that leaving the fresh juice of the berries on one's teeth for about five minutes and then rinsing with warm water which contains a small amount of bicarbonate of soda, will tend to remove discoloration from teeth. A great thing for herbalist who drink a lot of herbal tea.

I have also learned that Strawberry leaves contain Salicylic Acid that are helpful in dealing with pain.

In the area of salicylates; I just read an article by Jessica Marshall, written for Discovery News stating that plants "make methyl salicylate, a volatile form of salicylic acid." This is sent through the air when the plants are stressed, such as cold or draught to activate the plants immune system.

Sometimes I feel that plants talk to each other a lot more than we think. Aren't plants wonderful? The next time they talk to you, let me know what they told you.

Wild Violets

Viola odorata

Living in Wisconsin, I would be remiss if I didn't take time to talk about this wonderful plant. It just happens to be the State Flower of Wisconsin.

The name of this plant is taken from the flower but there are wild violets with pink flowers and some with white flowers. Mrs. Grieves, author of A MODERN HERBAL mentions that the word Violet when broken down is a deviation of via or wayside. These plants tend to grow in areas that allow the eight inch plant to thrive without much competition.

The Violet flowers always attracted my attention. I knew that they were edible and that they have a sweet taste in their base but until I read what Dr. James Duke said about them, I didn't think they had a lot of medicinal uses. A couple of the things that Dr Duke talked about was that they could be used for varicose and spider veins. This is so exciting because a lot of people that I know are dealing with this very problem.

According to Dr. Duke, "Violet flowers contain generous amounts of a compound called rutin, which helps maintain the strength and integrity of capillary walls." The amount would be a half cup of fresh violet flowers, I guess that is why I like eating them and get my 5 to 10 flowers a day. Dr. Duke mentioned that one could eat as many as 100 flowers a day without any adverse effects.

Mrs. Grieves mentioned that, "Piny prescribed a liniment of Violet root and vinegar for gout and disorder of the spleen. She states that a garland or chaplet of Violets worn about the head will dispel the fumes of wine and prevent headaches and dizziness." That sounds like a prescription for a good old fashioned hangover.

Violet flowers have been used in cooking for a very long time, both in the dish and as a garnish. I have used Violet flowers and find that most people pass them up instead of eating them. Maybe they just don't know what is good for them?

They have been used as a coloring agent and in the making of perfumes. They can also be candied as a dessert. A "Syrup of Violets" was made and was considered to be a nice dessert when added to lemon syrup or ice cream to be served in the summer months.

To get the best flowers from the plants means that they need to be thinned from time to time. When overcrowded, they tend to just grow a lot of leaves. They will also go to leaves when the soil is very rich.

A salad can be made by adding Violet leaves to any of the other garden greens. This salad might relieve a degree of pain as Violet leaves contain Salicylic Acid although not to the degree that can be found in Willow Bark or even Honeysuckle leaves. In fact, when I checked my resources, I found about 25 to 30 constituents contained in this little plant. Just think of the organic choices that one is giving the body when Violet leaves are included on the menu. When it is organic the body can use it or not as it wishes. When the body is given inorganic matter, it doesn't have those choices.

I read that one could cook the roots of this plant for food, so I decided to try that. The article suggested boiling them like potatoes. This was a very interesting experience as the roots have a slight bitter taste to them due to the alkaloid content. In the future I would cook them like acorns and do several rinses or changes of the water as they are being cooked. I have since read that medically the roots are used to incite vomiting. "They have occasionally been used as adulterants to more costly drugs, notably to ipecacuanha."

A tincture of the whole plant has been used for spasmodic coughing and Mrs. Grieves mentions that it can be used for rheumatism of the wrists.

We have deer that come into our yard mainly for the apples or the acorns but they also trim the tops off the Violet plants that are under the apple trees. Do they know something that we don't?

The leaves have been used to cure cancer. I believe the story goes that a nurseryman ate Violet leaves when he found out that he had cancer. He ate a lot of them and his cancer was cured.

Recently one of my friends asked me if we are responsible for all the cancer around us. I didn't have an answer at the time but when you look at all the things that nature provides us with to handle this very problem, my answer is, "Perhaps." Why the "perhaps"? I think it is because we keep eating the same foods over and over and over without taking advantage of what is really available to us. Violet leaves are wonderful for glands as a tea and even an ointment. When our glands are working the way they should, errant cells don't have a chance.

As you can see Violets aren't just for show. They might be shy plants but they do pack a punch.

Wood Betony

Betonica officinalis

Here is an herb worthy of being in everyone's medicine chest. Wood Betony is a small plant that grows in Europe. I will have to see about getting seeds or a plant to keep in my garden window as it produces pink flowers on long stems coming from the shorter plant. The leaves of this plant are scalloped and a bit hairy but what this plant can do will amaze you.

I learned about this plant during a phone conversation with another herbalist. She mentioned that she had to hang up and get some Wood Betony as she had a headache. My first thought was that I would use something else for a headache but when I did my research on this plant, I was convinced that this was the right plant to use.

Wood Betony has been handling problems of the head for centuries. I read where the Greeks proclaimed that it would treat "No less than forty-seven diseases", this according to Christopher Hobbs in his book called *STRESS*. Hobbs also said that it was a "Valuable tonic and nervine". This means that it doesn't depress the nervous system as many of our medicines do but will furnish the building blocks to remake or heal the area that is in trauma. When was the last time you fed your nerves?

Last night my husband came to the kitchen to get an aspirin. I asked him what was going on and he said that he had a headache from what he thought might be a stiff neck. He mentioned that it has been bothering him all day. That told me that he had been taking aspirin all day to *try* to deal with this. I allowed him to take his aspirin and then told him that I would like him to take a dropperful of

Wood Betony tincture before he left the kitchen. He wanted to know why? I told him that the aspirin would block the pain but that the Wood Betony would calm and rebuild the area that was creating the problem. In our society, we want to get rid of the symptoms before we have handled the problem. It would be like shutting off the door bell and not answering the door. The symptoms are the road map to the problem.

Wood Betony, as previously mentioned is great when the body is in stress. My tincture is fast acting. When you take a pill, it has to be processed through the intestinal walls but when you take something in alcohol; it is absorbed through the stomach walls making it "fast acting."

I want to list the things that Blake put into his Globalherb V2.0 computer program. He shows Wood Betony as being good for: anxiety, Cancer, congestion-general, cough, cramps, fatigue, gout, diseases of the head, headache, headache-chronic, hysteria, insomnia, intellect, jaundice, Migraine, Nervous disorders, nervousness, pain, Parkinson's Disease, senility, sores, swelling, twitching, and worms. You will notice that this list contains problems of the head but also other problems that a body can have from jaundice…a liver problem to cramps…a muscle problem.

I read in Hobbs book, STRESS, where people valued this herb so highly that there is "an old Italian proverb" , it says to 'Sell your coat and buy betony'.

The next time you have the chance to do something organic and natural for yourself, try Wood Betony.

Wormwood

Artemisia absinthium

This plant got its name due to its ability to expel round worms. There are a large number of members that fit into the round worm category. According to Hanna Kroeger's book PARASITES, THE ENEMY WITHIN, she lists; Ascara lumbricoides (common round worm), Hookworm, Strongyloides, Ancylastoma, Whipworm, Toxocara canis, Pinworm, Dirofilaria immitis (dog heartworm) Trichinella Spiralis as all being round worms.

Round worms are not the only kind of worms that humans can draw in to their bodies. Hanna has listed three kinds; roundworms, flatworms and single-celled parasites.

As mentioned in the first part of this article, Wormwood is wonderful at cleaning out (expelling) round worms or all the types that I have listed in that catagory.

Wormwood is very bitter and is usually not given full strength but in a combination with other herbs. While working at the herb shop, we would combine Black Walnut tincture, Cloves and Wormwood combination to deal with this. The Wormwood Combination is a creation of Kroeger Herbs and they have combined; Black walnut leaf, Wormwood herb, Quassia bark, Clove bud, and Male Fern root.

Hanna talked about parasites as being most misunderstood. When we go to the doctor and take a stool sample, he will more than likely find nothing. These parasites are cyclical. They are most active around the full moon. She suggested when trying to rid oneself of parasites, start five days before the full moon and continue ten days after. Then discontinue the program until five days before the next full moon and repeat. She said that the herbal treatment will rid the body of any adult parasite with the first treatment but before they are gone, some of them leave up to 30,000 eggs to be hatched at the beginning of the second round.

Recently I saw a television program (fiction) where a person had a parasite like this in their brain. That isn't so far-fetched; it is just that the media is starting to use this information. I have heard of breast lumps removed only to find parasites living in balls in the tissue.

Wormwood has other uses. Dr. Christopher talks about it being good for promoting digestion and correcting stomach disorders. He mentions that it will expel gas. It has been known to "counteract the effects of poisonous plants such as hemlock and toadstools."

Due to its bitter taste it is also helpful for the liver and will corrects things like jaundice. Dr. James Duke was right when he said, "Bitter is better."

Dr. Christopher mentioned that when taking a tincture of Wormwood, one must take it in a cup of water and in small amounts each time.

When I tell people that they have parasites, a lot of them are in disbelief. Parasites have a job to do in this world. It is their job to clean up and break down things that need to be recycled.

So when working with parasites, it is a good idea to remember than something is disintegrating before our eyes and maybe it is time to change the program and rebuild the body from the ground up.

We need clean air, clean water and good food, add to that a few different herbs from time to time to get a variety of nutriments into the body, and there just won't be room for parasites to live.

Hanna Kroeger told us that all things are vibrational in nature. She has many remedies to deal with the different kinds of Parasites, these remedies work from a vibrational level. If the vibration of the area changes, then what lived in that vibration, no longer has space.

Yarrow

Achillea millefolium

Yarrow is a Native American plant and the references that I found show that local Indians used it extensively. They called it "wound medicine" because it was so good for cuts, bruises, and other minor injuries. Because of its ability to stop bleeding, it was given the nickname of "nosebleed" by the white settlers for this reason. According to Dr. Christopher (Christopher – Volume 4 No. 11) the Micmac and Illinois tribes used it on cuts while the Winnebago Indians made a tea of it and washed bruises. The Thompson Indians of British Columbia powdered it by roasting the leaves and stems until they were dry, then ground them with stones and used the dust for skin sores.

The Indians of the Southern United States chewed the leaves fresh or dry with a little salt for a stomachache.

Eagle Shield, a Sioux healer, had some songs that he chanted when he was treating someone with Yarrow. It is no secret that Eagle Shield kept it in a very special bag as it was a sacred plant to him.

The warm tea is a diaphoretic. It stimulates the blood, opens the pores and causes sweating. This eases the kidneys by helping to get rid of the toxins fast while easing chills, fevers, colic, gout and also helps the liver.

When my husband comes home and tells me that he feels a cold or flu coming on and feels chilled, I serve a cup of hot Yarrow tea. I use four or five dried leaves in a cup and pour hot water over the top. It has a mild flavor but can be combined with a sweetener like licorice root. The next day I ask him how he feels and he can't remember feeling poorly, since the symptoms are gone.

In Dr. Christopher's "Cold Sheet Treatment" one starts with hot Yarrow tea to not only stimulate the system but to start the sweating action and hydrogenate the cells. He says that hot, wet fevers are safe and can get very high without damage. Hot, dry fevers are damaging to the brain.

As herbalists, we work *with the body* in helping it cleanse out the toxins; we do not take something to stop the action such as aspirin when we have a fever. The body creates the fever to handle the pathogens. If we stop the action, we are thwarting the body in its natural action. Pathogens live in a very narrow comfort zone. When the body takes itself out of its comfort zone, the pathogens leave or die. A fever is the body's way of changing the environment. When you have a fever your body is working at its very best. Help your body by drinking quarts of hot teas and soaking in hot, steamy water. After an hour of this, tuck yourself into a cozy bed and sweat it out. I did say drink quarts, didn't I? Yes, I meant it because your body needs all of this liquid to dispense with the heat it produces to kill its enemies. Help your body heal you. With this approach, I have known people to make a very bad flu last only 24 hours instead of the two weeks that they would have had to endure if they had hindered the process.

The GOBALHERB program says that Yarrow has about 90 constituents in it. Dr. Christopher credits them as dealing with: Fevers, eruptive diseases (measles, chicken pox, small pox, etc.), hemorrhage of the lungs and bowels, jaundice, piles, incontinence of urine, typhoid fever, diarrhea, colds, suppressed urine, scanty urine, wounds, ulcers, colic, diabetes, Bright's disease, stomach gas, relaxed throat, sore nipples, flatulence, congestive headache, and loss of hair. I would say that was a long list for one small plant to tackle.

The warm Yarrow tea is also a good eye wash, but make sure that you strain all the particles out first.

As a warm tea, I mentioned that it is a stimulant but as a cold tea it can become a tonic for convalescents. As a tincture it is used to decrease a heavy menstruation.

Some herbalists believe that it lowers blood pressure. The information that I found was that it does, but very marginally and there are betters herbs for this.

Yarrow might be something that you would like to grow even though it is found in meadows and along paths in the wild. Yarrow is a biannual plant. The first year it forms a mat of fern-like leaves where as the second year it grows upright on a single stalk with feather-like leaves. At the top of the stalk is a cluster of tiny flowers. When I imported some tiny wasps to deal with my gypsy moths, I was told to put these near tiny flower clusters. They loved the Yarrow flowers and because of all the botanical "fun" that is happening presently, one can find Yarrow flowers in many colors. I have a pink variety in my yard but when I am in the wild, I find white or yellow.

The crushed leaves have a unique smell that says Yarrow. I harvest the stalks and strip the leaves and flowers to be dried. The stalks have been used for centuries by the Oriental as a divining tool in I-Chi.

Yellow Dock

Rumex crispus

While riding in the car one day, I insisted that my husband stop so that I could find out what that brown plant was. (They usually get between 2 to 4 feet tall.) I got out of the car and found that it was a stalk of funny shaped seeds. Now I wanted to know who these seeds belonged to. I asked but most people have no idea what is growing around them, so it was time to research.

Did you notice that I wanted to know "Who" the seeds belonged to? Each plant has its own personality and is there for us to use. It is the human that needs to approach the plant because they have for a very long time felt we didn't appreciate them as beings.

I really learned a lot about this wonderful plant. The reason that I only saw the seeds was because the leaves had died off already. These leaves look strange as they are long, sometimes as much as 18 inches long and as wide as 2 to 3 inches. The edges of the leaves are wrinkled like stretched crepe paper.

The seeds have "wings" on them and grow on the top of the plant.

I used to think that this plant, being one of the docks like burdock was good for only its usable iron but after researching it, I have found so many good things that this plant is capable of doing.

I decided to see what Dr. James Duke's database could tell me and was amazed at all of the abilities in this plant. I decided to check on the constituents in Yellow Dock's roots. I will lay out some of the abilities that Dr. Duke attributes to these constituents. The following are capabilities in Yellow Dock roots: they are; Antiacne,

Antiaging, Antialzheimeran, Antianemic, Antiarthritic, Antiasthmatic, Antibackache, Anticapillary- fragility, Anticarpal-tunnel, Anticataract, Antichilblain, Anticolitic, Anticrohn's , Antidandruff, Antidementia, Antidepressant, Antidiabetic, Antiflu, Antiinflammatory, Antiinsomniac, AntiLyme, Antilymphonic, Antimaculitic, Antimigraine, AntiMS, Antipapillomic, Antiparkinsonian, Antiperiodontitic, Antipoliomyelitic, Antipsoriac, Antiseptic, Antistress, Antistroke, AntisyndromeX, Antitumor, Antiulcer, Antivertigo, Antiviral, Beta-Blocker, Cancer preventive, Candidicide, Cardioprotective, Hypoglycemic, Laxative, Pesticide, Spermigenic, Vasodilator, along with being an Antidote for lead and aluminum.

I wrote all of these out so that you can see how many things this one herb is capable of working on. Most of the time when I write that an herb is capable of doing this or that, I know that anyone reading has no idea of all the thing that it can do so this time I decided to show a lot of the information that I gleaned from the Database.

How do herbs do all of this? They do it by giving the body what it needs to handle the problem. It doesn't care what the problem is but if it has the ability to help in some manner, it will. Most plants will handle many situations. This is why I tell people not to just take one herb for whatever they are working on. Every time one ingests a different herb, we are giving the body more choices to use to make the corrections.

Dr. Duke has looked into all of the properties in this one plant and has mentioned that if one of these things is the problem, Yellow Dock might be able to provide what is needed to correct this situation.

I found that Yellow Dock Root has calcium available for the body's use. It also has chromium, iron, magnesium, manganese, niacin, potassium, protein, selenium and zinc. Most of all it acts like all the other Docks as a blood purifier and perhaps that is why it can take on so many things.

According to Duke's article in PETERSON FIELD GUIDE - MEDICINAL HERBS, the anthraquinones in this plant are great at arresting growths of ringworm and other fungi.

The root is said to be a mild laxative and this is probably due to the action it causes with the liver. A lot of Laxatives do work this way by making the liver release more gall into the bowels, thus relieving the liver and helping it to recover from its overload. (Gall being a good Laxative.)

One must remember that the liver is the detoxer for the entire body. Its job is to detox not only what we take in by eating or drinking but the toxins that we bring in through the lungs and skin from the environment. Now add to that the neurotoxins that we create with stress or anger or even hormones that we are releasing into the system. All of these things create an overload on one's liver.

Dr. Duke does have a warning about Yellow Dock that I will pass on, "Large doses may cause gastric disturbances, nausea, diarrhea, etc." It is *not* poisonous but again I wish to remind you to use herbs as foods. Just as you wouldn't eat a whole pie, you don't want to over indulge in any food/herb.

References - Part One

Baroody, Theodore A., N.D., D.C., Ph.D., C.N.C., **Alkalize or Die,** Holographic Health Press, Waynesville, NC, Eighth Edition 2002

Blake, Steven, **Global herb - Computer program**, version 3.0, California, 1995

Bremness, Lesley, **Eyewitness – Handbook – Herbs**, Dorling Kindersley, N.Y. 1993

Christopher, David, M.H. & Fawn, **A Healthier You – Audio Newsletter,** Christopher Publications, Springville, UT., 1999

Christopher, John R., Dr., **3Day Cleansing Program, Mucusless Diet, & Herbal Combinations,** 2002 Edition, Christopher Publications, Springville, UT., 1969

Christopher, John R., Dr., **School of Natural Healing**, Christopher Publication, Springville, UT.,1976

Clark, Hulda R., Ph.D., ND, **The Cure For All Cancers,** New Century Press, San Diego, CA., 1995, 590 pg.

Crow, Tis Mal, **Native Plants, Native Healing – Traditional Muskogee Way,** Native Voices – Book Publishing Co, Summertown, TN., 2001

Culpeper, Nicholas, **Culpeper's Complete Herbal & English Physician,** Meyerbooks, Glenwood, Il., Original printed in 1814

Duke, James A., Ph.D., **Dr. Duke's Phytochemical and Ethnobotanical Database,** 2003

Duke, James A., Ph.D., **The Green Pharmacy**, Rodale Press, Emmaus, PA., 1997

Foster, Steven and Duke, James A., **Peterson field Guides- Easter/Central Medicinal Plants,** Houghton Mifflin Co., New York, NY, 1990

Grieves, Mrs., **A Modern Herbal**, Dover Publications, Inc., NY, 1971

Hobbs, Christopher, L.Ac., **Stress & Natural Healing**, Interweave Press, Inc. Loveland, Co. 1997

Hoffmann, David, M.N.I, M.H., **An Elders' Herbal,** Healing Arts Press, Rochester, Vt., 1993

Hutchens, Alma R., **Indian Herbalogy of North America**, Shambhala Publications, Inc. Boston, MA. 1973

Kloss, Jethro, Reprinted with permission from **Back to Eden**, Lotus press, P.O. Box 325, Twin Lakes, Wi. 53181. © 1999 All Rights Reserved

Kroeger, Hanna, **The Basic Causes of Modern Diseases,** Hay House, Inc. Carlsbad, CA. 92018, 1984, revised 1998

Kroeger, Hanna Rev, **God Helps Those That Help Themselves,** 1984

Kroeger, Hanna, Ms.D, **Parasites-The Enemy Within,** Hanna Kroger Publications, 5th Printing, Boulder, CO. 1991

Mowrey, Daniel B., Ph.D. **The Scientific Validation of Herbal Medicine,** Keats publishing, Inc, New Canaan, CT. 1986

Murray, Michael. T., N.D., **The Healing Power of Herbs,** Prima Publications, Rocklin, CA. 1995

Olsen Cynthia, **Essiac- A Native Herbal Cancer Remedy**, Kali Press, Pagosa Springs, Co. 1996

Pedersen, Mark, **Nutritional Herbology,** Wendell W. Whitman Co., Warsaw, IN., third printing, 1995

Petrak, Joyce DCH, **How To Remember Bach Flower Remedies,** Curry-Peterson Press, Warren, MI., 1991, Revised 1992

Pollan,Michael, **Omnivore's Dilemma,** Penguin Books, USA, 2007

Ritchason, Jack N.D., **The Little Herb Encyclopedia**, Woodland Health books, Pleasant Grove, UT, 1995

Simonetti, Walter, **Simon & Schuster's - Guide to Herbs and Spices,** Simon & Schuster, New York, NY. Translated from Italian by Arnoldo Mondadoir, 1990

Tyler, Varro, E., PhD, **Herbs of Choice**, Pharmaceutical Products Press, N.Y., 1994

Index

A

abscess 24
Acne 24
alkaline 4, 33, 34, 35, 87, 89, 110
allergies 24
Aloe 96
Aluminum 38, 39, 52, 125, 140
anemia 45, 50, 58
angina 66, 76
antacid 4, 30
Antiacne 52, 139
Antiaging 45, 52, 117, 140
Antiallergenic 52
Antialzheimeran 52, 60, 140
antiarrhythmic 60, 82
Antiasthmatic 52, 60, 72, 124, 140
Antibacterial 18, 37, 41, 52, 55, 60, 79, 82, 88, 105, 109, 112, 114, 117, 119
Anticancer 18, 26, 55, 95, 114, 116, 117
Anticarpal tunnel 140
Anticataract 52, 60, 72, 105, 119, 140
Anticoagulant 101
Antidementia 52, 119, 140
Antidiabetic 18, 52, 55, 60, 72, 105, 114, 119, 140
Antifungal 15, 26
Antihistaminic 37
AntiHIV 18, 20, 60
Antiinflammatory 18, 20, 37, 52, 55, 63, 76, 88, 109, 112, 114, 119, 140
Antiitching 41
Antileukemic 52, 60
AntiLyme 140
Antilymphonic 60, 140
Antimalarial 72
Antimigriane 52, 57, 140
Antioxidant 18, 52, 82, 112

Antipapillomic 72, 140
Antiparkinsonian 52, 60, 72, 140
Antiperiodontitic 140
Antipolomyelitic 140
Antirhinovirol 37
Antisalmonella 109, 112
Antiseptic 14, 52, 60, 140
Antispasmodic 18, 30, 32, 38, 60, 89, 119
Antistreptococcic 112
Antistress 52, 55, 140
Antistroke 60, 140
AntiSyndrome-X 109
antitumor 26, 60, 63, 82, 140
Antivaginitic 116
Antivertigo 140
anxiety 10, 133
Appendicitis 10
Aromatic 30
arthritis 3, 24, 45, 50, 58
asthma 31, 40, 45, 47, 50, 57, 71, 83

B

bacteria 11, 33, 34, 52, 91
bed wetting 119
Beta-Blocker 140
bleeding 26, 34, 88, 113, 114, 125, 136
blisters 50, 123
blood xi, 10, 14, 16, 18, 22, 32, 33, 34, 36, 38, 40, 47, 48, 50, 54, 55, 56, 63, 65, 69, 71, 85, 93, 99, 100, 101, 104, 111, 112, 113, 115, 124, 125, 127, 136, 138, 140
boils 6, 24, 40, 45, 94, 102
bones 67, 69
Breast cancer 101, 103, 104
Bright's disease 137
bronchial 31, 40, 119

bruises 26, 39, 45, 71, 136
burns 10, 26, 40, 45, 73, 97, 116
Bursitis 24

C

calcium 7, 8, 15, 18, 38, 42, 47,
    65, 69, 72, 73, 84, 86, 87,
    98, 103, 140
Cancer 24, 26, 39, 40, 45, 52,
    58, 71, 103, 104, 122, 133,
    140, 143
Candida 11, 121
Candidicide 18, 26, 112, 117, 140
capillaries 67
capillaripotective 119
Cardioprotective 18, 26, 60, 112,
    122, 140
cellulite 40
Chaparral 93
Chickenpox 24, 31
cholesterol xi, 8, 40, 55, 65, 66,
    111
chromium 7, 38, 47, 52, 55, 65,
    140
circulation 19, 39, 71, 81, 94,
    108, 109, 111
citric-acid 7
cobalt 38
colds 31, 39, 40, 58, 71, 106, 111,
    137
cold sore 80, 102
colic 18, 39, 58, 99, 111, 136, 137
colitis 29, 39, 40, 44
collagen 67
Complete Tissue 44, 45, 86
constipation 5, 39, 40, 127
cramps 18, 35, 39, 82, 87, 133
Crohn's 29, 39, 40

D

dandruff 24, 74, 124
deafness 40
depression 9, 10, 20, 57, 58, 82,
    118

Diabetes 54, 94, 137
Diaphoretic 71, 110, 136
diarrhea 5, 39, 45, 58, 73, 75, 76,
    137, 141
digestion 4, 6, 10, 32, 55, 90, 135

E

ear 10
eczema 24, 40
Edema 24
Essiac 22, 143
estrogen 12, 13
estrogenic 13, 18
expectorant 44, 71
eyes 34, 40, 41, 82, 111, 124, 135

F

female organs 48
fertility 82
fever 5, 6, 39, 40, 45, 58, 114,
    137
Fibromyalgia 124
flavonoids 67, 103
flu 24, 26, 31, 37, 58, 61, 103,
    106, 136, 137
fractures 45
frostbite 10
fungicide 15, 26, 52, 60, 63, 119

G

gall bladder 5, 50, 82
gangrene 39, 45, 74
gas 29, 30, 31, 39, 49, 135, 137
gastric ulcers 39
gastritis 39
generative organs 82
Ginger 97
Gonorrhea 24
gout 24, 40, 45, 103, 125, 127,
    129, 133, 136

H

hayfever 40, 45

heart valves 76
hemorrhoids 26, 40, 88, 114, 116, 125
hepatitis 50
Herpes 24, 79, 80, 90
high blood pressure xi, 18, 50, 127
hives 37, 78
Hollyhock 76
Horsetail grass 68, 69, 87
H. Pylori 33
Hyperglycemia 24
Hypoglycemia 24, 50

I

Impetigo 24
incontinence 137
indigestion 39, 58, 103
infection 14, 40, 41, 77
inflammation 11, 24, 39, 45, 48, 55, 57, 95
insect bites 6, 51, 58
insomnia 10, 133
iodine 14, 84
iron 6, 7, 8, 14, 18, 38, 42, 52, 103, 105, 115, 124, 128, 139, 140
Itching 24

J

jaundice 20, 26, 39, 48, 71, 133, 135, 137

K

kidneys 6, 20, 44, 48, 83, 111, 136

L

lactating 55
laxative 28, 83, 92, 140
Leprosy 24
liver xi, 5, 6, 8, 9, 20, 24, 26, 37, 39, 44, 48, 55, 60, 63, 65,
71, 124, 127, 128, 133, 135, 136, 140, 141
Lobelia 5, 84, 85, 87
Lung 10, 55, 83, 114
lymph 26, 84, 85, 124
Lymphatic congestion 24

M

magnesium 6, 7, 15, 18, 38, 42, 55, 65, 103, 124, 140
manganese 7, 38, 42, 52, 55, 140
marc 53
Measles 137
menses 20, 26, 32, 63, 82
menstrum 53
Migraine 57, 58, 133
Milk Thistle 65
mosquitoes 40
MSM 59
Muscles 10, 19, 28, 81, 108

N

Nausea 57, 141
Nerves 19, 20, 30, 59, 118, 119, 132
Nervine 30
nervousness 39, 133
Neuralgia 18
Newcastle Disease 90
niacin 7, 38, 42, 52, 55, 72, 140

O

Oatstraw 87
obesity 40
Omega-3 96
oxygen 6

P

palpitations 18, 66, 81
pancreas 48, 50, 103
Parasites 15, 88, 103, 117, 134, 135
phosphorus 7, 18, 38, 42, 103

phyto-hormones 12, 13
plaque 66, 80
pleurisy 40
Poison Ivy 24, 123
Poison Oak 24, 123
postpartum 82
potassium 6, 7, 14, 15, 18, 38, 42, 47, 65, 103, 115, 124, 140
pregnancy 18, 32, 102
prolapsed rectum 88
protein 7, 38, 42, 80, 140
psoriasis 24, 40, 58
pyorrhea 26, 86

Q

Quercetin 55

R

Rashes 10
Refrigerant 30
Relaxant 32
rheumatic arthritic pain 35
rheumatism 18, 24, 40, 71, 110, 127, 130

S

Scarlet fever 24, 31
sciatica 24, 118
sclerosis 71
selenium 7, 14, 38, 47, 52, 65, 140
Shingles 41
silicon 18, 38
Silver 5
sinus 34, 41, 55, 87
skin 10, 19, 26, 32, 33, 36, 37, 38, 40, 41, 48, 50, 54, 60, 67, 73, 74, 75, 76, 79, 83, 86, 88, 96, 101, 103, 110, 119, 124, 127, 128, 136, 141
Smallpox 24, 31
sodium 6, 38, 84

Sodium fluoride 84
sore breasts 45
sores 24
sore throat 19
spider bites 51
sprains 26, 45
Staph 94
stings 10, 16, 41, 77, 123, 124
stomachache 24, 136
Stomach problems 90
Stomach ulcers 34, 114
stroke 48, 107, 108
strong teeth 67
sty 24, 41
Sulfur 103
swelling 26, 39, 45, 77, 88, 94, 95, 133
Syphilis 24, 26, 101, 111, 127

T

teeth 67, 86, 97, 119, 128
Tendons 67
thiamine 38
thyroid 13, 14, 84, 85
tin 7, 38
tincture 16, 19, 21, 37, 51, 52, 53, 62, 80, 81, 88, 111, 114, 120, 130, 133, 134, 135, 137
tonics 107
tonsillitis 24
toothache 26, 39
torqued muscles 108
triglycerides 55, 65
Tuberculosis 76
tumor 24, 104
typhoid fever 114, 137

U

ulcerations 27, 58
urinary tract infection 77

V

vaccine 72, 90

varicose veins 88
Vasoconstrictor 18
Vasodilator 18, 52, 60, 63, 112,
      119, 140
Vitamin A 38, 42, 72, 105
Vitamin C 38, 42, 65, 67, 72
Vitamin K 125

W

warts 14, 27, 83
water retention 24
weightloss 50
Whooping cough 101

Z

zinc 7, 38, 42, 47, 52, 55, 140

Part Two

The World of Spirit

Jumping right in, I would like to tell you how I found my way to the spiritual world of plants.

It all started with a book called "The Magic of Findhorn." Well, of course I would gravitate to a book that has the word "magic" on it as you can see by the title of this book. I wanted my world to be more magical and full of wonder.

In this book about three people in Scotland who built a community under the directions of nature spirits, I found the "magic" that I was looking for. Peter and Eileen Caddy along with Dorothy Maclean were the main characters of Findhorn. The author had heard about this wonderful community and wanted to know how it was done.

The garden that they used to sustain the three of them was grown on Scotland's sand but with the help of Spirit and Nature, they were able to produce large quantities of food. Some of the produce was oversized and that attracted the attention of the world.

It seems that Eileen would meditate and get instructions from Spirit on what they should do and how to do it. Peter said that it was his job to implement what was told to them. Dorothy was the one that connected with the Devic kingdom and relayed their messages. (Deva is a Sanskrit word for "Being of Light.")

This book excited me even more when Peter went to London to talk to his friend, Crombie, who was able to see the nature spirits of the parks and talk with them. At first when Crombie made contact, the spirits wanted nothing to do with him but little by little they started talking to him. He told Peter that they could communicate when he showed no fear.

Once he was sitting by a tree in the park and a nature spirit came up to him playing a flute. When Crombie talked to him, the spirit was very surprised that he could see them. In the course of all of this, the man even invited one of the nature spirits to his flat. He showed this spirits his extensive library and the nature spirit couldn't believe that humans needed all of this to "know" things. The four-foot high nature spirit told this man that all information is available to everyone, everywhere. Nature spirits didn't need books to know, they just knew.

In the late 1980s, Peter came to Wisconsin to speak at an alternative community near Plymouth. One of my co-workers wanted to know if I would like to go with her. We went. We both came away with different ideas. She was disappointed with the old man that she saw. She wanted to know why he wasn't tackling his next project. I think she expected him to go from one major accomplishment to another. People don't do that. Sometimes we have just one large project to accomplish in this lifetime. Peter had done that. He had helped create a wonderful spiritual community in Scotland and help create a large awareness of co-creating with nature and Devas. I saw a man who had created a masterpiece and it was continuing under the direction of other people. (Findhorn is still a wonderful retreat center in Scotland.) I was impressed with what he had put together and wished him bliss in his old age. I was hooked by the creations and ideas presented in this book and knew that I had to find this in my life.

I grew up in a wooded area in northern Wisconsin. Even then I knew that when I was in the woods, I was not alone. But how to find the beings that I felt around me was my quest. I would spend hours under a pine tree or sitting on the branch of a tree about 10 feet off the ground. I would put an arm around that tree, I thought I was hanging on but when I think back perhaps the tree was holding me? That tree looked out over the lake and it knew my darkest secrets. When I was in trouble, my mom knew just where to find me...in the woods, in my tree.

I recently purchased some herbal "Throat Soothers" from St. Claire's. Debbie, the founder of St. Claire's, has something written on the inside of the cover of this purchase. "The secret of making something work in your life is, first of all, the deep desire to make it work; Then the faith and belief that it can work; then to hold that clear, definite vision in your consciousness and see it working out step by step, without one thought of doubt or disbelief," by Eileen Caddy." Now to put this into practice in my "can do" world.

Dorothy Maclean, a member of the Findhorn project, later wrote about the Devic realms that she found while living there. In Dorothy's book TO HONOR THE EARTH, she talks about the spirits of trees, air, mountains and according to her, just about everything has a guardian angel. She quoted from some of them about their areas of responsibility. The Devas of the fruit trees told her, "Nothing is worth doing unless it is done with joy; in any action, motives other than love and joy, spoil the results. Could you imagine a flower growing as a duty and then sweetening the hearts of its beholders?"

That is such a wonderful thought that even reading it makes me breathe a sigh of relief. It seems so important for the whole earth to be tended by loving beings put there by GOD.

One of the things that Dorothy said she learned from the Devas was their suggestion, "That I learn to think in terms of inner forces by looking at all forms as made of light, glowing and radiant." She also found that Devas are a joyful group and "radiate love to everything without judgment."

Dorothy also states, "To me their main theme was not how to grow gardens or how to understand life but the injunction to attune to the uniqueness of our souls and accept and act on the powerful love in our core."

This is heavy duty stuff and most people have not even the slightest idea what she is talking about.

Years ago I was told that I had cancer. It was a frightening time for me but through this, I met LOVE, my friend or Guardian Angel that is with me. I nick-named him LOVE. He was shaped like a capsule about four feet long that radiated yellow/white light in every direction. It was a very bright light but one could look directly at it as it was really unconditional LOVE. After this encounter, when my physical tests came back, the doctors couldn't find any cancer. You have heard it said that if you are still here on Earth that means your work isn't done. Well, I knew that my time here wasn't but I wondered if the LOVE being would stick around. He has, by the way. I never walk alone.

I have always had an affinity for plants so that is where I was directed. It seems that every place that I have lived needed someone to put it together with LOVE and I had him with me to do just that. I think anyone can send unconditional love to others. When there is a problem, I breathe in Unconditional Love and direct it with my mind to where this Love should go. We all know that love shouldn't need to be directed. If one is balanced and working with a LOVE being, one should be able to radiate this to everyone. That has been the source of some problems as when people feel this projection of love coming in their direction, they want more. It seems that they think I have their answers too. At times I have found that people feel taken care of and don't want to stand up for themselves but for the most part it has been the source of great joy.

Books started coming in my direction like, THE LOST LANGUAGE OF PLANTS by Buhner. He talked about how plants communicate chemically with us, and with each other. Some of us don't understand the words that plants use, but that doesn't make the communication less valuable. Some people just get feelings instead of words. Some of these chemicals come in as smells and will brighten our days. Buhner talked about healing some of his clients with the language of plants. He told about healing a lady when she made a connection with Angelica, a plant that loves water, has large leaves and the stems are hollow. He had her breathe in the language that Angelica was telling her, after which he watched her whole body change before his eyes.

THE SPIRITUAL PROPERTIES OF HERBS by Gurudas was another book that looked interesting. It was so exciting to find others that had looked in the direction that I was now searching. These books talked about some of the experiments that have been done on plants to see what they are capable of doing. It was talking about the way herbs are handled and signature plants (Plants that look-like what they are used for.) Gurudas listed a few herbs that had a "high" spiritual value. I just knew that I was headed into some exciting stuff in these books.

In between books, I found classes of various forms. My uncle wanted to attend a class but didn't want to go alone. It was called the Silva Mind Control Class. He was told by his doctor to quit smoking or die and this class advertised the fact that they could help one control habits. So we went.

The Silva method helps you learn to use more of your mind. What was it that Einstein said, that we only use about 10 percent of our ability. I found this class very interesting when our homework one night was to have a pad of paper by our bed and every time that we come close to waking up; we were to jot something down on the paper. When it was almost morning I heard one of my children call out "Mom" so I jotted this down and shook myself awake enough to respond. What I found when I was fully awake was that someone had let the dog outside last night and didn't let him in. He was at the back door barking. Wow! I can interpret "dog language" now. I had to laugh at that but there it was on my pad of paper. "MOM" and all my children were sound asleep.

It was at the Silva classes that I got introduced to my Female Guardian Angel. I told you about LOVE coming to me when I was physically in trouble but in this class they mentioned that we would meet our angels. I went to the instructor and told him that I already had one and didn't want to mess this relationship up. He told me to go through the guided meditation and see what happens.

Well, you can imagine when my male guide appeared, I was very nervous, but it was LOVE who walked in. I was so happy that he was still with me, that I remember thanking him for being there. When my female guide was to appear I wasn't sure what to expect. Then another four-foot capsule came forward. This one was transparent but you could make out the edges of her egg-shape because inside of this being were sparks of different colored lights flashing from one side to the other and bouncing back all over in different directions. She was beautiful. I just stared at her. I saw so much energy bouncing around that I decided to nick-name her ENERGY. I never was told her real name, but I could have called her Beautiful because that is the way she looked. (I have to admit that LOVE did tell me his real name but I have continued to call him LOVE anyway.)

The next book that pulled me in was titled BEHAVING AS IF THE GOD IN ALL LIFE MATTERED by Machaelle Small Wright. The first half of this book was her biography. It was interesting and traumatic but I wanted to get to the good stuff. When was she going to talk about the "GOD in all life?" About half way through the book, I hit pay dirt. Here she told how she met the Nature Spirits and how to communicate with them. I was elated. This felt so right... Machaelle Wright!

She talked about the Devas of things like Carrots and how the plant angels pull in what that seed needs to make it what God intended. She talked about how to co-ordinate a garden so that everything works together. One of the things that I thought about while reading this is that when one creates a garden, one is creating an orchestra as each seed that is placed into the ground sends out a sound to draw the Deva of that plant to it. Each sound is different so one wouldn't make a garden of all carrots. It would be like only having violins in the orchestra. One needs to create a harmonic garden, where the sound of each plant creates harmony with the rest of the plantings.

I liked what Machaelle had to say. Somewhere inside of me, it made so much sense. I remember when she talked about garden bugs and how to deal with them. She didn't spray the garden with some chemical but rather she talked to the Deva of the bug, (Yes, they all have them) and told it that they could have one plant of their choosing. When she came out the next day, only one cabbage had caterpillars on it and not in abundance but only what that plant could handle. Yes, this is my kind of gardening!

A few weeks after finishing her book, I had an experience that you can read about later in the article, "The Apple Garden." I hope you will enjoy reading it and see what happened on my first try with all of this. It was and still does amaze me.

Many years later, our 100-plus year old oak tree was covered with gypsy moths. They were heading west and the Politians were trying to hold the line on this side of the Mississippi. Nature never did listen to people rules. We didn't want to lose the oak tree so my husband and I were trying different things. I called the parks people to see what they could do and as I don't allow spraying on our property, they couldn't help me.

The first thing that I did was put a four inch band of molasses around the tree. Our tree took two bottles full. It did slow the caterpillars up a bit so I could pick them off but that didn't handle the problem. (I usually don't kill bugs either.) I contacted some people who suggested importing some parasites. I found a place out west that would send me some tiny wasps that lay eggs on the caterpillars and the immature wasps would eat the caterpillars. The people from the parks department were really upset because I had introduced a foreign parasite into the area. (They had no problem spraying and killing lady bugs or any other beneficial parasite.)

Finally I called Machaelle Wright's research center called Perelandra, LTD in Virginia. The first thing that they told me was to STOP WARRING! They suggested that I ask the tree what it needs to handle this and what the Gypsy Moths need to stay healthy. Then allow *them* to work it out. That was a few years ago and we haven't seen any since but then the State has still been warring so perhaps they have done aerial spraying.

One of my friends gave me the book SILENT SPRING by Rachel Carson which talked about how we are poisoning our planet with chemicals. Carson spoke about when the Fire Ants and Gypsy Moths invaded the east coast of the US and the amount of spraying that was done that killed so many birds and small mammals along with all the beneficial bugs. I believe that she felt about the chemical companies as I feel about the medical community. Carson took on the chemical companies because she had a scientific degree. Makes me wish that I had a medical degree and could rebel again all the chemicals pills that are being shoved into mankind but the people who do this lose their medical license. I will continue to try to get through to people on an herbal level.

Most books that I read having to do with plants and gardening are so uplifting that I come away feeling great. Reading SILENT SPRING made me ashamed to be human and my soul cried for this planet.

The next event that came into my life was a lecture by a man named Michael J. Roads from Australia. I decided to attend his lecture after all I must be headed forward to have a *Wright* and now a *Roads* in my life. (Can't get better sign posts than that.) His book is called TALKING WITH NATURE. In this book he quotes nature as saying that it is time for humans to get acquainted with Nature.

He said that for him this came about as the results of a plant seminar that he attended near a grotto. He knew that he needed to return to the grotto alone and when he did, nature opened up. "*Be*

Welcome. By no accident are you here. People from many aspects of life find their way to this pool. It is a place where barriers are laid aside and defenses dropped. It is here that many people are able to 'feel' the essence of Nature for the first time."

His lecture was so wonderful. He talked a lot about the continuum of life. How one life feeds other lives and how all things are connected. He had us role playing as the rabbit and how it continues to run even after the fox has it in his mouth. The spirit of the rabbit keeps going. It kind of makes me think of a skier who hits a tree and leaves the body there but continues down the hill.

Of course his book was my next text. This is my training field. While talking to nature, he writes how nature thinks that humans are very limited. *"Your words are true about your limitations, even if they are self-imposed and therefore not real. Within our kingdom, light shines with undiminished purity.... Such illumination reveals to us our place in the design of life."* Wow! And here we are all looking for that, a direction and plan for ourselves.

My next adventure was to attend some hands on healing classes, similar to Reiki (Energy healing). In this class the teacher talked a lot about energy. We would take turns being worked on by four people, one on each side of us, one at our head and one at our feet. The people on the sides moved our energy around to stimulate the organs and to get the chakras moving (Energy centers in the body.) The person at our head blew energy into the top of our head. The person on our feet would pull off the energy and ground us into our bodies.

As a painter, I found myself seeing colors around people while we were working on them. One evening our teacher took us into an empty room with very little light and told us that we were going to look at auras or the energy that is always around each of us. I remember seeing the smoky colors around these people. After that the other students wanted me to tell them what color they were that night.

As we finished the series of classes, the teacher suggested that it might be nice for me to do some automatic writing. I had no idea what that was so she explained it to me. I was to have a pad of paper and a pen, then go into a meditative state and ask questions that I wanted answered. You will read more about this in another article.

Learning more about plants was the next direction for me. I wanted to know what they could do and how they did this. I attended a class given by Rev. Hanna Kroeger (a nationally known herbalist) on the medicinal uses of plants. I was so excited about what she said that I was ready to roll up my sleeping bag and go to Colorado to learn everything she knew. Of course that wasn't possible because I have a family that expected me to be here but when she gave week-long classes, there I was. I have notebooks full of what she talked about. Some of the things that she would say were so far beyond my believability at that time, that I would just shake my head and write it down. When I go back into my notes today, they aren't that unbelievable. So if I hear someone talk about their carpal tunnel problem, I immediately think of Hanna and hear her saying that here is a person who is not being appreciated enough.

Hanna told us about all the herbs that could be used for this and that. She taught us how to get answers to our questions with a dowsing tool. When I tried to dowse with a pendulum, it was like picking up the phone and getting all my questions answered without any doubts on my part. Maybe this was because as a child, I watched my grandfather use a split willow stick to find artesian wells, three to be exact. Who were we connecting with? Spirit!

I wanted to learn more about the medicinal uses of plants and how they worked. Hanna just told us what worked. I talked to a friend of mine and she suggested The School of Natural Healing in Utah. I decided to check out a few herbal schools and found out that the founders of a lot of present time schools had studied with Dr. John R. Christopher at his school, The School of Natural Healing so I decided to do that. I came away from those lessons with a new understanding about healing and a new understanding of using plants to do this. I started to teach some classes in my home for people who wanted to know what I had learned. This was not in the realm of Spiritual learning but I know that Spirit wanted me to do this. I have always felt guided in my life and we learn even more by teaching.

The spirits are always around us. There are times when someone is having a major problem and I am doing fine so I will ask LOVE to go to them and help them in their time of need. Most people have been raised in a specific religion, so did I but this seems to fit with everything that I had learned. Why wouldn't a loving God supply us with assistance, both on the physical and the spiritual level and help us to understand all of it?

My next step came from one of my students. She brought me a book and told me that she thought I would be interested in it. The title of the book is THE ELVES OF LILY HILL FARM by Penny Kelly. Like most people, Penny had this wonderful experience and kept it to herself because she didn't want people to think that she was different. That happens a lot when you step out of the norm that is walked by most people. Penny didn't know how to fit this into her world until her husband told her it was time to put it out to the public.

The Kelly's run a working farm in southern Michigan. They grow organic grapes for Welches. She decided to go back to school and get a counseling degree to help people like us to find our way without the judgments that are out there. The farm has turned into both a working farm and also a learning/counseling center.

After reading her book about working with the "little people" I tried to find her on the internet. I wanted to write to her but I only found one reference to her and it was wonderful. The internet brought up farming information. The first article was about a man in Wisconsin who grows Apples using the method that the Kelly's use to grow grapes. I have a feeling that the "Elves" told her how to do this. In both cases, they have speakers placed in the field/orchard and do sonic blooms in the field.

According to what I read in the back of Penny's book; "Sonic Blooms" is: "A registered, trademarked system of plant nutrition that combines special sound frequencies and a rich organic nutrient sprayed on the plants." She also has a "Sonic Doom" and it is: "A registered, trademarked system of weed control that combines special musical frequencies and minimal amount of herbicide to eliminate weeds without saturating the soil with poisons." It seems that the parasites on the grapes don't like the noise/sounds either. I guess that goes for Apples too.

The Kelly's sell organic grapes to Welches for the Juice that you get to drink. Hanna talked about using specifically Welches purple grape juice in lieu of a blood transfusion. She had a few other things that could be used to increase the blood and make it healthy but I will not be mentioning them here. Hanna felt that by putting other people's blood into your system, you were doing more harm than good. Our blood carries our DNA/RNA so by taking on my blood you would inherit all the problems that have been handed down to me.

Penny talks about how the "elves" first came to her, not in her first book but in the second book, ROBES - A BOOK OF COMING CHANGES, she opens up and tells all about her first real encounter with the "Little men in brown robes." They talked to her about everything from the dangers of present-time chemical medicine to the changes that are headed this way for the whole planet. It is my perception that the second book happened in her life before the first one but she was afraid to write about it. It was at the nudging of her husband that she opened this up to the world.

When she encountered the little people and could communicate with them, her world changed. Everything on her farm was subject to the Devas and the Elves.

Here I would like to explain that Devas and Elves are quite different. Devas are the spiritual side of the Nature world, but Elves are independent beings that seems to live in a dimension that we are not always aware of. When dealing with a plant, one would contact the Devic Realms. Elves seem to have territories that they tend. That is to say, they look out for the flora and fauna of their area. Most of us find these interchangeable.

I decided to take a gardening class at this time and the University Extension had one that sounded great. The pamphlet said that they wanted to teach gardening using the smallest amount or no chemicals. Now they were talking my language. The classes were great on how to physically garden. I was told over and over again that I was not allowed to talk about the medicinal properties of any of the plants. By this time I had studied with the School of Natural Healing and gotten a Masters degree, making me a Master Herbalist. I didn't understand their resistance to my talking about plants and their healing properties but then it dawned on me. Our

University gets most of its money from Drug Company research so of course they didn't want me talking about how these plants could be healing. I had to resign.

Recently I have been introduced to the Ringing Cedars books. It is a series of nine books that have been written in Russia about a Siberian recluse who communes with God and nature on a very personal level. These were written less than 10 years ago and talks about the need for people to return to the closeness of nature for health and wellbeing.

While reading one book in this series, I took time out to record all of one chapter on the proper way to plant seeds and seedlings to have them respond to your individual health needs. It seems that nature wants to be our doctor by drawing into it what each individual might need to correct the imbalance in our bodies.

What intrigued me was how we can introduce ourselves to each seed, a seed containing the potential of the plant, and then the seed will draw to it what I need for healing. Having worked with the Devic Realm, it was easy to imagine that instead of this seed sending out the sound of middle C, it might send out a C sharp so that the Devic realm knows that it needs more of this or that. Isn't that an exciting idea?

Most people reading this would think that all of what I talk about is imagination because in their worlds it is. However, when one walks in more than one world at a time, life takes on a new dimension. The book that I am reading right now tells me that our reality is shaped by our thinking. What we think, we can create after all we were created in the image of GOD the supreme creator. So if you want men from Mars in your life, they will be there and real for you.

It just so happens that I want everything in my life to revolve around nature and this planet.

As you can see in these writings, I am always being shown something different and more exciting. It is like LOVE and ENERGY just know what I need next in my growth process. So when someone suggests something, I jump in with both feet. In this way I get to decide if it fits into my life or not. Some things don't fit but I won't know that unless I take the time to look. One of my biggest pet peeves is when someone has judged something without ever trying it on to see if it fits.

What do you want in your world?

Co-creating with Plants

In the course of learning about plants, I found that they like our energy and they like to be given time to assimilate information. If a tree is to be cut down, a three-day notice is required for the spirit of that plant to leave. I know that most of you will find this strange but we need to treat these beings as our brothers, remembering that without them, we cannot breathe. It is time that we start to respect all living things. We have not been doing that for a very long time but then again most people that I know even take their close family relationships lightly.

Recently, we have been having long periods of drought in our area. Not to the point of losing plants yet, but where a lot of little things like Wild Ginger and my mints are drooping. In Penny Kelly's book, ROBES –A BOOK OF COMING CHANGE, she said, "Trees and vegetation are other critical elements in moderating and controlling electromagnetic fields, and therefore the wind. Trees are themselves producers of magnetic fields, and their fields interact with magnetically charged pockets of air and land in two main ways.

One is that they keep air moving through sheer intelligence. Trees are intelligent beings capable of shifting the electromagnetic signature of the E-M fields they produce. Thus, they are capable of attracting air pockets containing moisture when they are dry and want something to drink."

After reading this, I told my large trees, Oak, Maple, and Locust, that they were not doing their job. They are supposed to bring in rain for the other beings around them. I gave them quite a talking to and to my surprise, within 24 hours, we got water. First, it was just a sprinkle, followed later by an all-day easy rain. Boy, did I feel foolish.

Then I had to go out and apologize to them. It didn't make any difference what the weatherman had to say about the situation, as they had been promising rain for a week but the trees really did it.

As a small child, I don't remember my parents having to water the yard, but then we lived near a lot of trees. My grandfather used to bring small cedars from the woods to our area to mark off the land. He built wind buffers with them and it helped keep the snow from drifting in some areas.

In the Ringing Cedar's books, the author Vladimir Megre talks about what the damage of having large farms did to Russia. It seems that with all the stable grasses cut down and farming with standard large farm practices (that means with chemicals that kill the micro-organisms and the natural bacteria in the soil) the large plains of Russia are starting to become deserts. The soil is not able to produce like it once did. Trees, along with old-fashion farming techniques are what is needed. This is why the Ringing Cedar series is pushing for people to set up their own little corners of small farms and incorporate a wooded area in each of these little farms.

We went through this when we dug up the central plains area of the United States to "feed the world." The plains were growing wonderful tall grasses and we came along with our "know it all" knowledge and created a dust bowl.

I read once where the southern part of France was desert-like until a lot of trees were planted there. Sorry, but I can't remember the reference on this. The point is that without trees to take care of this planet, it will not take care of us.

Co-creating means to work with nature. We need to find out how we can do this. We need an awareness of nature. I hear people telling me, "It is just a tree." And my heart cries because their awareness is so small. I am appalled when I see Christmas trees. This is a very old German custom to cut down a living being for our amusement and celebration. Then I am told that it gives employment to many people. I heard that same thing about nursing homes. At one time I knew that there was a better way to deal with elderly people than warehousing them but I was told, "It gives people employment." What a sad commentary. We need to see the big picture. We need to learn to co-create.

A few years ago, I went before the planning commission of our area to thank them for not making the eighty acre wooded area north of my property into another soccer field. Most of the time when they are given land they make it into a park that has a playground and a baseball field and a few soccer fields. But in this case they left the area wild with the exception of some trails through it. Lately they have added a few benches to sit on.

Nature spirits are all around when one goes into a wooded area that hasn't been anything else for a very long time. In the woods north of us, there is a part of it that has a very high canopy of Oak and Maple trees, with a lot of small bushes under it. To sit in this cathedral of trees surrounded with trillions of spiritual beings, rivals any church in the world.

This area that I am talking about doesn't seem to need fertilizer to stay healthy. It doesn't need to be weeded to be healthy. In fact, I think it is better off than if man were to come in and carefully plan everything.

I took a gardening class and they tell me that when I want to plant a seed or small plant, I need to do this in "Sterile" soil. I have never understood that. None of the small plants in this woods even knows what sterile soil is. And if I kill all the micro-nutrients in this soil, what will my seed live on? I could buy some chemicals I suppose but I don't believe my plants want that. I can check with them and let you know.

Machaelle Wright talked about how the Devas supplied what her garden needed. She mentioned that once she was told that she needed to put some straw or something like that on a portion of her garden. She wasn't sure how she would get what was needed but later someone had driven past her driveway and accidentally dropped what she needed. She mentioned that she had no way of knowing who it belonged to as no one came back to pick it up. You don't suppose that the Devas helped it fall off a truck?

I do know that my seeds and small plants like to be given energy. One can do that by talking to the plant but I like to create a ball of energy and give it to each individual plant. They tell me that they can use my energy like sunlight/food. I am happy to hear that. This can be done for seedlings and to plants that have been recently trimmed.

I do it to my house plants in the winter time. In the summer they are put outside to commune with the sun, moon and planets of the sky.

It is my belief that we were **not** given dominion over, but were put here to co-create with nature. We have not been doing that for a very long time. Maybe some of the good books need to be rewritten?

Feelings

If one talks to my husband about feelings or even wants to talk to him about feelings, he isn't interested. But if you ask him what he thinks about something, now you have a discussion.

Why are people afraid of their feelings? All of the people that connected with the Devic Realm, started by connecting with feelings. I would get a feeling to do this or that and by following through, I found that it would work.

Let's just take one situation. We had a family party at our house and one of our relatives had recently died. The person closest to that member was going through the grieving process and hadn't dealt with everything yet. There was a lot of turbulence in the group. When everyone left, I *felt* that the energy in the house needed to be cleaned out.

There are many ways to clean energy out of an area but my choice at the time was to imagine a pink wash over everything. (I do watercolor painting) I started in one room and with my hands brushing the air and my vision of "pink", I brushed the walls, the furniture, and the ceiling with a pink light. I continued to do this until the whole house had been cleaned. It took on a very different feeling. Later my Devas told me that it had been a good thing to do.

How many times have you done something and you get the feeling that it was the right things to do? Sometimes people tell me, "What you just said, made my hair stand up." Which is another type of feeling that a lot of people use to confirm something to themselves.

Once my sister wasn't feeling well; I told her that she could come and spend the day on my couch or be at home alone. She decided to be at my house. As she slept, I *felt* that we needed to burn the problem out. So I collected as many candles as I could and set them on the end tables, floor and anywhere else in the room that would hold them. When all twenty of them were burning, I sat back to make sure that she wouldn't wake up and have to run over any of this while on her way to the bathroom. When she woke up, the first thing that she wanted to know was, "Did I die?" She wasn't ready for this but the problem was gone and the candles were blown out. (By the way, most of my family has gotten used to my doing things based on *my feelings*.)

Another time my husband wanted to have someone come to our property to aerate it. I guess I didn't understand just what that was because this young man came with this large-loud machine and walked all over the property as fast as his legs could take him. The plugs were flying in every direction. I started to cry, I felt the pain. All over my body, I felt painful pricks. My skin hurt. Someone had just violated my corner of this planet. He had with no feelings at all as he pulled up plugs of Gaia's skin.

For the next two days with tears running down my face, I collected these plugs and put them in the compost pile in the back yard to be recycled back into our area. I ordered some topsoil and put it into each hole. I kept apologizing to the planet for this crude act of violence toward her. She told me that it would be all right but the fact that I cared so much was really the healing factor. I mentioned to my husband that if he ever wanted to do anything like that again, the person that is hired has to agree to hum or sing while doing it so that it isn't a violent aggressive act.

Feelings are just another language that we use to communicate with everything around us. When a person wants to know what herb to take for what is going on in their body, if they would just take the time to feel/listen, they would know what they needed. Most of these plants have so many abilities that even if they took the wrong herb, it would do its best to help the situation.

While I was rollerblading with my daughter, I fell. Then knowing that I had damaged my body, I went inside and looked around to find all the damage. I could communicate with all my parts to know what problems needed to be dealt with. I broke my arm but was anything else in trouble? Each cell will communicate if we take the time to listen and feel what is happening.

We expect people outside of our bodies to know what is wrong with us.

When I go outside on a warm summer's night, I sit on the grass and *feel* the energies around me. If the Devas wish to show themselves, I am entertained by a light show. Some of these beings of light are larger than other. Some are just little sparks. They come in colors too but they aren't visible unless they *feel* wanted.

Sometimes I feel that I need to be the connector of energies. I will stand on my yard making an X out of my body. The energy of the sky is transferred through me to the ground and vice versa. The best thing is that these energies cross each other in my solar plexus. Everyone benefits.

Today while driving home on a country road, the car in front of me slowed down because a dog was out there chasing and barking at the tires. I reached out with feelings and words and told the dog that this isn't what he wants to do and he left before I got up to that place in the road.

We have all been somewhere when we get a feeling that we need to leave and get out of there. We know that we are being warned. What happens to people that don't get those feelings?

One time I had a feeling that I needed to do a blessing on our property. I went to one corner of the land and with arms outstretched, I thanked God for the trees, the land and the beings that live and visit our property. Then I asked God to bless every living thing that resides here or visits it, to give them the feeling of welcome and joy. Then I went to the next corner and did the same thing. At the third corner, the man across the street told my back that I look funny doing that. I just continued. It is okay to look funny. From there I went to the forth corner and did the same blessing. I finished with a big "Thank you God!" All from a feeling.

The next day, our area had a flood and water was all over the neighborhood. We joked about having lake front property because the water was coming up on the back yard and running across the driveway. The house next door had 3 feet of water in the basement. I had a pile of sand so we used pillow cases to sand bag around their basement windows . The house that the man who spoke to me lives in was running two sump pumps to try to keep his basement dry. We didn't get any water in. All of this from a feeling!

I had a tabby that used to sit on my shoulders to look at my pictures while I read. Cats are really good mind readers and they like the pictures we make as we read. At the time I was reading all of Jean Auel's books that talked about a primitive woman who made friends with animals.

This same tabby would come up on my lap and without using her claws; she would swat my face if I were crying about something.

There were times that I *felt* like I was crying for the whole world. I didn't have a problem at that time so it wasn't me that I was crying for. My girlfriend told me that I probably was crying for the planet as so much was happening at that time. All of this was long before Global Warming was even known by anyone. Okay so sometimes being sensitive to the world around us can be detrimental but at least, if we know what it is all about perhaps we can help?

Feelings are not bad things. People who live without utilizing their feelings are missing half of what this world has to offer. It is all right to open up and allow intuition and feeling to help you navigate in this world. The next time you are around an animal or a plant, check in with feelings and find out a little about their world, maybe they will introduce you to their angels.

The Apple Garden

Our house is on a corner lot where two streets meet. At this corner of our property, live two apple trees. They were planted in a set of three by the previous owners but one of them had died and was still standing there when we moved in. The dead tree was removed and the area mowed cleanly.

Mowing around the remaining two trees was a problem for my husband so I decided to create a small garden area under them. My first thought was to decide what I wanted to create. I decided on a football design with the area between them being wide and ready for some planting.

It was Spring and time to begin the digging. The temperature was in the 40s so I bundled up and headed out. First I dug around the area to do a layout. Then I started to take the grass off the inner part of my design. These clods were tossed onto the yard and I spent most of the morning clearing the designated area. The design was perfect.

Then I had to get the area ready for plants. I had purchased a creeping Juniper to keep the corner low and visible for traffic in all directions.

First I dug up the ground and then dump a couple bags of peat and composted manure on the area. Now the best part, I got to mix all of this in with my hands. The soil was just right; it was like mixing biscuit dough. As I was mixing, I would throw the stones that I found out onto the lawn with the grass clods. Soon it was all mixed in. I stood back to admire the work that had taken me a long time to do and to my surprise, I found that there were energy waves rising from this little garden. They look like heat waves coming off black top roads in July and it wasn't that warm out.

I felt that I had to do something so I ran into the garage to get a slab of cement and brought it out to the little garden. After placing the cement between the two apple trees in this newly mixed dirt, I went around the whole garden picking up the little rocks and stones that I had thrown onto the surrounding grass. These stones were placed on this cement in a pile.

When I stood back this time, the energy had been grounded and the garden didn't look like it is about to float off into space. I was pleased with all of it and it was time to plant the Juniper.

The little garden looks wonderful and has done its job of keeping the lawnmower away from the base of the apple trees and the branches from knocking my husband off the little tractor.

Before I started this project, I had read a book called BEHAVING AS IF THE GOD IN ALL LIFE MATTERED, by Machaelle Small Wright. In this book she talks about communicating with the spirit guides of plants. I wrote to her and told her about this experience of mine and she wrote back telling me that she was pleased that I responded to the spirit guides nudging me to ground the garden. She explained that most people just read about this stuff but never do anything with it. It seems that these thoughts and feelings that we get are not always ours but help from other areas or beings.

Over the years this little garden has been enlarged bit by bit to encompass the trees as they grow. The garden also has a lot of wild violets living there along with some chickweed that I harvest. There is a lot of love and energy in that little garden and it tends to draw deer to it from the woods that are about half a mile from our house. The deer come in the spring for the violets. They love violet leaves. (I have been told that violet leaves are very anti-cancerous, I wonder if the deer know this?)

There is Chickweed that I like to harvest for all of its wonderful drawing properties. A few years ago some Columbine decided to live there and because I like their flowers, I leave them growing there. I do plant flowers on the street side of the garden, I like Calendula because I can harvest the flowers and the plant still puts out more. They aren't fussy plants and don't mind being neglected from time to time.

The Apple Garden gets visited by the deer in the fall. They like the apples and are allowed to eat them. This year we donated the apples to some horses that belong to a friend of mine.

From time to time, I climb into the apple trees to trim the sucker out. What is the saying about apple trees? A bird should be able to fly through the center of the trees. This allows the sun and air to get into the trees and keep the trees healthy. I used to have a bird house in one of the trees but if finally fell apart. I really like bird houses and have only 3 on the premises at this time, will have to look into that. I do have a bee house in the apple trees at present so I probably won't put a bird house back there.

We have many small gardens in our yard and they all have their own names. The Apple Garden was an obvious name for this one. One of the reasons for the small gardens is that I can have a variety of things and yet I don't have a lot of work. This week I might tend one garden and then next week a different one. Having small gardens doesn't overwhelm the gardener.

Gardening is such a pleasure, one of the joys of life and a way to connect with Mother Earth and listen to the spirits of nature.

Trees that Heal

When we tend to carry more than we should, we feel it in our backs. What in fact happens is that we have muscles on both sides of our backbone, and when one side gets tense; the other side gets pulled out of place, thus a back problem.

Recently I had been carrying more emotional junk than I should so my upper back "went out." I headed for the woods. Walking slowly and bent over, I walked up to the first very large tree that I came across. I leaned my back against the east side of that tree and told it that I need some healing. I remember mentioning to the tree that it only needed to give me a little because I would visit other trees in the forest.

The east side of any tree is very healing. Wendell Hoffmann, author of several books talked about using the energy of a tree to heal a lady who had breast cancer. Using copper wire, he connected her to the east side of a tree for a day. The next day he came back and did the same thing. After three days of using tree energy, she had no breast cancer. (Referenced from Using Energy To Heal by Wendell H. Hoffmann page 79)

After thanking the first tree, I walked very slowly through the woods and found another large tree. I repeated what I had done the first time.

After that it was time to sit on one of the downed trees and be grateful for the energy that was all around me. When one is alone in the woods, the energy is a very powerful feeling. There is very little negative energy in the middle of a woods. Perhaps that is why so many people are angry, they have lost their connection to this energy, this life force? They are depending only on their personal belief system, while continuing to function in the middle of the negative-energy pools of other people.

After doing some communing with nature, it was time to walk on. Some of the plants had already lost most of their leaves this fall. Some of the leaves left were so orange, pink or yellow; it flooded the eyes with a feast of color. I remember complimenting a 2-foot maple on the gorgeously colored leaves that she still wore. I asked if I might have one. She was a very proud maple as I accepted a large orangy colored one. I thanked her with the hope that she continues to grow without interference from animals, which includes the other people that will pass by her in this forest. Along with the leaf, I found a feather and that always is a sign that I am welcomed. Single feathers are gifts that always make me smile.

Having made most of a circle in this woods, I came across a very large oak tree. As I leaned up to it, I told it that I only needed a little healing and pointed out the spot that needed attention. I stayed there for quite a while comforted by the feeling of that beautiful big tree. We had connected so when I left, the discomfort was gone from my back and I no longer walked slowly or bent over.

For those of you who have never connected with a tree, I would like to tell you that it is different than anything you might think. Each tree has a different personality, much like people. I have been told that each species of trees has a different personality.

One time I asked to be connected with the Deva of the Oak tree on our property. (Deva is a Sanskrit word for Being of Light) I was told that it might be overwhelming, as it is the largest spiritual being in our area.

Old Oak trees have a way of overwhelming a person. Their personality is that of a wise old soul. They get right to pertinent information. The first time that I talked to a tree, I jokingly said, "I bet you know the secret of life?" And to my surprise it replied, "The secret of life is to make a place of peace and comfort for those around you." They all do this but Oak will tell you this right up front.

Maple trees, on the other hand, always seem to be joyous, comfortable and bubbling over with happiness.

Before I could leave the woods that day, I had to give thanks for the gifts that they had given me, not only for the healing but for the nourishment of my soul. All Plants have a way of doing that even when you're not ready.

The Others

What would you like to ask, if you could get an answer to any question that you have been thinking about?

When I was taking a healing class in Racine, we would work as a group on different members. Each time we met, everyone had a change to have some part of their body worked on. Yes, it was energy healing. We had learned to pull "junk" out of the area that we were working on and help move energy up and down the body. Whoever was working on the feet would pull the energy down and off the end of the body. Our teacher mentioned that people tend to live in their heads and sometime we find that their spiritual feet have pulled up to their knees. We have to anchor them back into their bodies. The person working the head area would blow energy into the top of this body. Everyone in the middle would work to keep the energy moving by keeping the chakras spinning.

One evening our teacher told us that she was going to show us what our aura looked like. In a darkened room, with only reflected light from a hallway, she stood by a white wall. We watched as she pulled up Mother Earth's energy into her body. Then she pulled down the God energy from the sky and combined them in her solar plexus area to be able to move this energy out of her hands. We watched her shoot swords of light to a wall five feet away, through her palms. I remember commenting that she was constantly changing color. She explained that the God energy is a different color than Earth's energy.

Once we could see the energy around the body, she asked each of us to come up by the wall and allow the class to see the energy around us. When it was my turn, I showed them how I make balls of energy and send them off. Usually I do this to plants but in this case I just sent these balls of white light to the nearest wall. Those who could see energy talked about it, the rest of the class was still learning.

Because most of the people there only saw the energy, some of them ask me what color they were. The colors seem to be colored smoke that floated around them. People don't come in one color but have different colors in different places on their bodies. For example, their arms might be light blue and the head might be yellow. I don't really understand the colors and what they mean but it isn't hard to see them, it just takes practice. We have to look with our spiritual eyes and not have any expectations.

My teacher suggested that I try some automatic writing. I had never heard of that before but why not. It did sound like something I would like to try. She told me that I should get into a meditative state, then ask questions and see what happens, being prepared to write it down.

My husband goes to bed at 8:00 pm summer or winter so that sounded like a good time to do this. After it got dark out and the house was quiet, I lite one white candle, and then relaxed in a chair with a pencil and paper on my lap.

I have found that when I meditate, I relax and wait for the "Colors". In my mind's eye, I see different colors that whorl around each other much like the colors in an oil slick. They just move this way and that way. I don't really concentrate on anything but enjoy watching the colors. I found this way of meditating when people would tell me to clear my mind of every thought and just allow. Every time that I "allowed" the colors would come.

Now to ask a question, at first I wasn't sure what to ask so I decided to ask about the Devas, the Plant angels.

My first questions was:

Q: How do I get more insight on Devas? Will they ever approach me?

There was a very long pause as I poised my pencil over the paper. Still not knowing what would happen, little at a time I would get a word and write it down. Sometimes waiting for the next word, I would imagine what it would be …but I usually got it wrong.

A: *It is all not known what you need to know. How would we share? We need together? We understand your limitations. We need others to be one. We see all in one in everything. There is no one only all. Time is only now. Form can change at will. The will of the designer. God is the designer. Many can redesign something. It will follow blueprint. We are helping it. Example, transfer. Normally more love on inside. Enlighten area. Caring and loving energy, they transmute into food. The plants use it like sun's energy. We are open, wish to share and guide.*

Wow! That was interesting. I don't understand it but…. So my next question was…

Q: Why is my Cat here?

A: *She is aware of us, is viewing this conversation.*

(Side note: when I was reading Jean Auel's books about the wilderness life of a primitive women, my cats would come to enjoy the pictures that I created in my head. Cats are very good at reading pictures.)

Q: May I talk to the Devas of Oakwell?

A: *You are there, we are all and share. Much stress on us too. Most are stressed. Send love/light at all times. Much stress. Many changes now and ahead. Many of us around you most of the time. People very unaware. We enjoy your energies. We are one, we share energies. We can try, we can share our oneness. We are here to help. Lighten your heart. Fill with love.*

Q: What can I share with my healing group that would be helpful?

A: *Things are on schedule.*

Q: what does that mean?

A: *Each person is where he is meant to be. All is well.*

Q: Why are we impatient?

A: *Think in fast forward not now.*

Q: Why do I have a headache?

A: *It is Vern's*

Q: It is also gone now. Thanks. May I talk to the Oakwell Devas?

A: *It surprised you to ID the owner of the pain. We too pick up that around us. Much pain, hurting. We get very sad. Have to let it go. We need less stress, noise, hurting. We feel human hurt, anger. It is hard on us. We liked the pink light you cleaned out with after the family party. It helps put balance into areas. When we are in balance we assist those around us. Chain reaction. We are able to put stop to bad and not pass that along. Do it by transmuting it. This takes energy. Light is wonderful. Pierces soul/heart. Check water tomorrow. Some help needed. Remember to lighten heart and send love. We are you.*

I waited a while and then because my cats were running around all over the place, I asked,

Q: Who are my cats chasing?

A: *The beings in this room. Many were drawn by your music and meditation. Most important to bring Christ light in.*

Q: What do you look like to my cats?

A: *Like little sparks of life. The God/good energy.*

Q: May I talk to the Devas?

A: *We are all here. We are all one. Many things to do. No time to do. Give all. Must find more time. We will help you understand it. Extremes are good. People need them to understand the middle. Value your judgment. Must be careful not to rush people. Most are rushing to catch up. The party allowed you to do the catching up. Need to see others that are just ahead of you. Time means nothing; it is all in the heart. We will bless all. Have heart smile. Give love.*

Q: Is there anyone or anything else I should know about?

A: *The light of the rose is beautiful, radiant. Send to everyone. Be there. Allow more. All are sparks of God, all are learning.*

(In my meditation I was shown a rose with light coming out of the rose from the base of each of the petals. I asked about it and was told that was how my soul looks to them. This can be very humbling.)

Q: May I talk to the Oakwell Devas?

A: *You can see why we play games with you at times. We need joy. There is joy only as it is created. All can create. The tapes are very good. All truth is everywhere. Send more love/light into areas. Be free to help all who need. You will be guided. We are here. Your light attracts us. We enjoy it. There is much light. All need it. Love to you. The heart is good. We are you.*

Every time I sat down to do this, I felt that maybe I was talking to myself. So I tried to see what words would come to me next because I would get one word at a time. So the next time I asked:

Q: How do the Devas feel about a plum tree?

And I got one word at a time again that said..

A: *We accept your triangle but would like to help.* (When I heard the "we accept" I had no idea how this sentence was going to be finished, so the rest of it was all theirs. They continued to say…) *All needs to be put together with love. All is not right. We need your input. We like fruits…Must give more thought to design when spring comes. All need redesigning. We will work together to have a co-created garden. We need you to see our ideas and do. Friend left to be part of celebration (*I told Vern a few days before that I thought there was a pine tree in the back of our neighbor's yard that was missing. When I was out there, the energy felt different.*) Only form left, being still resides in the pines. Apple area needs cooperation. Pear not happy with area. We will work on that. Send love even in the winter. We will care for all. All are one. Love heart. We are you.*

I did this through the winter of '92-'93. What I put down here is verbatim of what I got during that time. Later in '93, I got a lot more information. Some of it relating to others, some relating to family situations but all of it telling me that I am here to help and that I have more resources than I am aware of. I don't always feel that way and yet I know that I am never alone. I have always felt that in this lifetime I am here to help the planet (and everything on it) to move into the fourth and fifth dimensions.

"And I saw a new heaven and a new earth, for the first heaven and the first earth were passed away." (Revelation) "For as the new heavens and the new earth, which I will make, shall remain before me, saith the lord, so shall your seed and your name remain."(Isaiah)

We Are All One

Isn't it interesting when all the things that you believe start to show their faces? Lately I have been finding this happening.

I enjoy watching the Public Broadcasting WORLD channel on TV and a few days ago they were talking about string theory. This is something that scientist have been working on for a while. The premise is that mass particles and waves are interactive. Let's see if I can put this a little simpler. According to what I understand, matter can be made up of particles and sometimes these particles turn into waves or vice versa.

While watching my favorite program, this lecturer was talking about turning gasses into liquid etc. I find that fascinating but then he mentioned the particle/wave idea and I sat up quickly. What did string theory have to do with this? He went on to talk about the Einstein Bose Condensate. This sounded interesting, something new for my mind to wrap around. (Learning is my erotic zone.) So what was this new idea? It was the fact that matter can be made up of particles and/or waves and sometimes when the waves have been altered a bit by extreme cold, *they become each other.* (He went into Absolute Zero, another interesting concept but this will wait until another time.) As one can see, I don't have the Einstein Bose Condensate theory down but I do understand this last part, *they become each other.*

They become each other, **is** the center of my life. It is a concept that I have been embracing for a very long time. When I would have weekly talks with the Devas of Oakwell, they would continue to tell me that *"We are one."* That could have meant that they are all joined together but I really think that they were trying to tell me that all beings, and now all matter is one.

That sure would fit with my concept of the universe.

I read a book called TURNING HOME by Paul F. Eno and in it he talked about all sorts of things but what hit me from that book was a Biblical translation that he quoted. I have never really felt that the Bible was translated the way it was written and he confirmed this. The quote that he used was Matthew 22:39. In the Bible it says, "Love your neighbor as yourself." Isn't that a beautiful thing to think about? But Paul Eno says that the original Greek that this comes from is," agapesis ton plaision sou <u>os</u> seauton." He even underlines the "os" in this. He said that the real translation is: "Love your neighbor because *he is yourself.*" And they become each other.

When you hurt, I hurt. When you are happy, I am happy. We are all one.

That really doesn't seem to fit into our world, does it? I am different from you. I am a certain political party member. I am a certain religious member. I am a certain race. I am....... But what am I really? I am you!

Will we ever understand that concept? What would happen if we did? Would we stop fighting? Do we need the separation to be ourselves? Are we afraid of losing our identity?

Yesterday a lady stopped by to chat. She was telling me about a long time friend of hers who just decided that they were no longer friends. The lady mentioned that maybe it was a good thing as they didn't have much in common anymore. They have life in common but it isn't always enough.

Why do people come and go in our lives? God created us in his image to experience life on this planet. Does that mean that we are each different? No, it means that we are all in our own experience of this life. We collect experiences and they shape what we think and how we feel about everything. Does that make us different? To the degree that each experience impinges on our soul, that would be a "yes".

I don't really know anyone who is not experiencing major trauma in some manner at this time. We are all being forced to learn. The climate in the world is about change, in all aspects and each of us is being forced to learn so that we can do this.

Many years ago, when I was finding myself being super sensitive to those around me, I would get a pain in some part of my body. It might be a headache or a pain in my knee. I found that by looking around at one of the people who was nearest me, then going inside my head and asking "Is this yours?", it might go away. If not I would continue my search. To test this out I would go up to that person and ask if they had a headache. They might say something like, "Does it show?" I would make up something to answer this with, "Your eyes looked dark. I just thought you might have a headache." (I don't get headaches) How about the knee problem? "You seem to be favoring that leg." I took on the physical problems of those around me. We are all one.

I had to work very hard to shield myself from the problems of others. We have been taught to shield ourselves from each other until we think.... Yes, we only think we are separate beings on this planet.

We are all one! Find yourself in those around you. We are part of the life force on this planet, we are all one!

The Magic of Life

Every place that I have lived has had its bit of magic. While living in Merced California, we moved into a small house on a lot that was fenced with a four foot picket fence. Actually it was a tract home and all of the houses basically looked the same. This tract was three miles out of town, on what had been farm land and not a lot had been done to the property.

The builders had put one tree in the middle of the back yard for everyone; ours happened to be a fruitless Mulberry. And when I saw it for the first time, the trunk was about two inches in diameter. (Mulberries grow rapidly) The yard was a combination of weeds, grass and sandburs.

With three small children that I wanted to corral in this yard, I needed to do some work.

I didn't know a lot about gardening or Devas or anything like that back then. What I did know a lot about was patience. As a child I had spend hours and days sanding boats with my dreams and a goal of having fun with that boat, I could do that here. I dreamed that this yard would be beautiful and a safe place for my children.

First, I dug all the way around the yard and put in a hedge of privet and flower beds. We installed a swing set near the back fence and a sandbox on the side of the house.

I put in a cherry tree near the east side and a plum tree in the back of the property. While digging up for the flower beds I found a Star Jasmine plant that must have been run over by the lawnmower many times because we had never noticed her before. Once I dug around her, she decided to become a beautiful plant. I also found a fruit tree about a foot high near the back fence, it turned out to be a pomegranate that had never had fruit. All of these treasures were given the attention that they deserved.

The lawn was the next thing. No one could go out there without getting full of sandburs. So every evening I would go out after supper and sit on the ground while pulling sandbur plant out of the yard. I would try to take a square yard of lawn and make it bur free. (They spread out but only have one root.) Now this is a lesson in patience if ever there was one but at the time it didn't seems to be a burden. I would listen to the children and watch them swing and play. It became a time of relaxing while sitting with my family.

I have always been a scrounger so when a house burned down about a field away, I went over there and brought home some slate that was being dumped out. This slate was then laid in a pattern under the Mulberry tree to make a small patio, with large potted plants put on it along with our old lawn furniture, making it a place to sit outside and relax.

As the yard continued to look more like what I saw in my head, I added a little Magnolia tree toward the back of the property. This was no easy feat. When I dug in where this tree was to be planted, the ground was rock-hard. I later found out that it is called hard-pack where the clay packs down and is almost like rock. I chipped and chipped and chipped through the six inches of this, finally I was back to good soil again. Now I could plant this beautiful tree.

As the Mulberry grew I built a tree house. This tree wasn't large enough to handle a "house" or small children in it so this "house" was a platform on four by fours that stood next to the tree. The branches were around the platform and the kids had a place to climb to and feel like they were in the tree.

After supper one evening, I was at the sink doing the dishes while my husband was sitting on the patio under the Mulberry tree reading or working out something. He was a realtor and liked to figure out the best way to help buyers close on a property. The kids were playing in the tree house and on the swings. It was one of those days when everything seems to be going right. The sky was somewhat clouded over but because it was toward evening, and the sun was low enough to send rays under the clouds at a wonderful angle. The back yard looked like a paradise. Everything was glowing in the light of this almost sunset.

I remember looking out of the kitchen window, taking everything in. I was thinking how everything seemed so unusually beautiful. The flowers that I had lovingly planted and watered were all smiling in the sunshine. The privet hedge that my farm-friend, Muriel had helped me put around the property, now formed a five-foot hedge and looked great. I had been trimming them to make a wonderful enclosure with them. The Cherry tree, while still only about 4 feet tall was in blossom. The Plum tree near the swing set was also in blossom and even the Magnolia, as small as it still was, had one large white flower smiling at me. I had worked very hard to create this garden and it was just the way I wanted it.   I found myself filled with love for everything that I saw. The feeling that I had was overwhelming. My cup runneth over!

In the next instant, I was 8 feet behind me on the other side of the kitchen. I knew that I was looking at the back of me because there was my long blonde hair and I was wearing a white blouse with blue slacks. I felt so frightened in that moment that in the next instant, I was looking down at my hands in the dishwater.

Wow, what had just happened? Things like this just don't happen in my world. I don't think I have ever heard any my friends mention something like this. What had I done to create this affect? I must have been doing something to make this weird thing happen? (This turned out to be one of the first unordinary things to happen in my world and I wasn't used to it yet.)

Let's back track. What had I been doing? I had been loving our back yard with the same kind of love that one reserves for people. Can we love things that way?   I had been loving the trees and the bushes and the patio and the flowers...everything because they looked so loveable. OK, so is that what Jesus meant when he said that there was only one kind of love? (I don't know if he really said that or not but this is what I was telling myself at that time.) I remembered something from church about three kinds of love but I don't believe that anymore. I can love a tree the same way I love my child. I can love a flower the same way that I love my husband. There is only one kind of love. This is big stuff! Unconditional Love?

I had to digest this for a while. A few days later I decided to see if I could create that situation again. Could I duplicate that intense love and pop me out of my body again? Why not try?

It took a lot to figure out just how to recreate that feeling, the intensity and the kind of love that I had witnessed. I kept adjusting the feeling and yes,... I could leave my body and view things from a different perspective. I could watch me doing things like talking or cleaning or relating to other people or just listening to them. What I found out was that I had to bring this love from deep inside of me then send it out through my eyes. It has to be very intense and unconditional, but it can be done.

Once, I wanted to see if a camera could pick this feeling up. As I worked on getting the intensity just right, the photographer asked me if something was wrong. I guess I do look strange but when that picture was developed, there were comments about it that weren't usual. One person many years my junior, asked the owner of the picture if I was married. Could one really send this love in picture form? I guess the answer is "yes".

Many times after that I would leave my body and go to another part of the room, watching how I was relating to whomever my body was near. Sometimes I found myself near the ceiling but not all the time. I would study what was happening, what my body language was and what was the body language of the person I was interacting with. It was a very interesting study. It felt like flying and swimming at the same time only with thoughts instead of movements. After a while it didn't seem to accomplish anything so it wasn't that much fun. I decided to not do it anymore.

What did I learn? Unconditional Love is very powerful when used right. We haven't even scratched the surface of learning about this. There are so many possibilities to explore. Life is Magic.

The Seed as Physician

The following information was found in the book ANASTASIA by Vladimir Megre. I have been given permission to reprint it in this book. I think it is vital information on how to work with nature for the benefit of our health. Sometimes what we think of as strange is really the most natural way of doing something. When we become set in our ways, they become unnatural.

This is an Excerpt from ANASTASIA by Vladimir Megre (pp77-81) translated by John Woodsworth, edited and footnoted by Dr. Leonid Sharashkin and published by Ringing Cedars Press (2005). English translation copyrighted© 2005-2008 by Leonid Sharashkin. Used by permission.

Anastasia has stated:

"Every seed you plant contains within itself an enormous amount of information about the Universe. Nothing made by human hands can compare with this information either in size or accuracy. Through the help of these data the seed knows the exact time, down to the millisecond, when it is to come alive, to grow, what juices it is to take from the Earth, how to make use of the rays of the celestial bodies – the Sun, Moon and Stars - what it is to grow into, what fruit to bring forth. These fruits are designed to sustain Man's life. More powerfully and effectively than any manufactured drugs of the present or future, these fruits are capable of counteracting and withstanding any disease of the human body. But to this end the seed must know about the human condition. So that during the maturation process it can satiate its fruit with the right correlation of substances to heal a specific individual of his disease, if indeed he has it or is prone to it.

In order for the seed of a cucumber, tomato or any other plant grown in one's plat to have such information, the following steps are necessary.

Before planting, put into your mouth one or more little seeds, hold them in your mouth, under the tongue, for at least nine minutes.

Then place the seed between the palms of your hands and hold it there for about thirty seconds. During this time it is important that you be standing barefoot on the spot of Earth where you will later be planting it.

Open your hands, and carefully raise the seed which you are holding to your mouth. Then blow on it lightly, warming it with your breath, and the wee little seed will know everything that is within you.

Then you need to hold it with your hands open another thirty seconds, presenting the seed to the celestial bodies. And the seed will determine the moment of its awakening. The planets will all help it! And they will give the sprouts the light they need to produce fruit especially for you.

After that you may plant the seed in the ground. In no case should you water it right off, so as not to wash away the saliva which is now covering it, along with other information about you that the seed will take in. It can be watered three days after planting.

The planting must be done on days appropriate to each vegetable (People already know this, from the lunar calendar). In the absence of watering, a premature planting is not as harmful as an overdue planting.

It is not a good idea to pull up all the weeds growing in the vicinity of the sprouts. At least one of each kind should be left in place. The weeds can be cut back..."

According to Anastasia, the seed is thus able to take in information about the person who plants it and then, during the cultivation of its fruit, it will pick up from the Universe and the Earth the maximum amount of energies needed for a given individual.

The weeds should not be disposed of completely, as they have their own appointed function. Some weeds serve to protect the plant from disease while others give supplemental information. During the cultivation time it is vital to communicate with the plant. And it is desirable to approach it and touch it during the full moon at least once during its growth period.

Anastasia maintains that the fruit cultivated from the seed in this manner, and consumed by the individual who cultivated it, is capable not only of curing him of all diseases of the flesh whatsoever but also of significantly retarding the ageing process, rescuing him from harmful habits, tremendously increasing his mental abilities and giving him a sense of inner peace. The fruit will have the most effective influence when consumed no later than three days after the harvesting.

The above-mentioned steps should be taken with a variety of plant species in the garden plot.

It is not necessary to plant a whole bed of cucumbers, tomatoes etc., in this manner; just a few plants each is enough.

The fruit of plants grown like this will be distinguished from other plants of the same species not only in taste. If analyzed, it will be seen that they are also distinct in terms of the substances they contain.

When planting the seedlings, it is important to soften the dirt in the excavated hole with one's fingers and bare toes, and spit into the hole. Responding to my question "Why the feet?" Anastasia explained that through perspiration from one's feet come substances (toxins, no doubt) containing information about bodily diseases. This information is taken in by the seedlings. They transmit it to the fruit, which will thus be enabled to counteract diseases. Anastasia recommended walking around the plot barefoot from time to time.

"What kind of plants should one cultivate?"

Anastasia replied:

"The same variety that exists in most garden plots is quite sufficient: raspberries, currants, gooseberries, cucumbers, tomatoes, wild strawberries, any kind of apple tree. Sweet to sour cherries and flowers would be very good too. It does not make any difference how many plants of each kind there are or how big their area of cultivation is.

There are a few 'definites' without which it would be difficult to imagine a full energy micro-climate; one of these is sunflowers (at least one plant). There should also be one and a half or two square metres of cereal grains (rye or wheat, for example) And be sure to leave an 'island' of at least two square metres for wild growing herbs – ones that are not planted manually. If you have not let any of them growing around your dacha*, you can bring in some turf from the forest and thereby create an island of natural growth."

I asked Anastasia if it were necessary to plant these 'definites' directly to the plot, if there were already some while growing herbs close by – say, just beyond the fence – this is how she responded:

It is not just the variety of plants that is significant, but also how they are planted – the direct communication with them that allows them to take in the information they need. I have already told you about one of the methods of planting – that is the basic one. It is essential to infuse the little patch of Nature surrounding you with information about yourself. Only then will the healing effect and the life-giving support of your body be significantly higher than from the fruit alone. Out in the natural 'wilds' (as you call them) – and Nature really is not wild, it is just unfamiliar to you - there are a great many plants that can help us cure all- and I mean –All – existing diseases. These plants have been designed for that purpose, but Man has lost, or almost lost, the ability to identify them.

I told Anastasia that we already have many specialized pharmacies which deal in healing herbs, just as there are many physicians and medicine men, who make a profession out of herb treatments and she replied:

"The Chief physician is your own body. Right from the start it was endowed with the ability to know which herb should be used and when. How to eat and breathe. It is capable of warding off disease even before its outward manifestation. And nobody else can replace your body, for this is your personal physician, given individually to you by God, and personal only to you. I am telling you how to provide it with the opportunity to act beneficially on your behalf.

If you make connections with the plants in your garden plot, they will take care of you and cure you. They will make the right diagnoses all by themselves and prepare the most effective medicine especially designed for you."

*dacha – a country garden

Foot note:
Please note that store-bought seeds available in America and elsewhere in the 'civilized world' are often coated with rat poison for ease of storage, and should not be used for planting in the way recommended here. If you wish to follow the planting advice set forth herein, be sure to use your own seeds or procure organic seeds from a reputable producer (available from many on-line and mail-order vendors or through health food stores.

I feel that this article would be helpful for those of you who want to start your healing gardens. We are looking at a time in history when regulations and laws will make it impossible for us to get the kind of health care that we need. As Bernard Rosen spoke about in the Foreword of this book, changes are afoot that require each of us to heal ourselves. When I read this article, I knew that it was something that each of us should know about. I wrote to the publishers and got permission so that we can create our gardens and let them help us become healthy.

Herbally yours,
Phyllis Heitkamp MH

Insects are Friends

While doing my chores today, the Devas told me to write about insects. They called them bugs because that is what humans call them. I asked why I should talk about that, they mentioned that it is because insects do not get appreciated. Humans love flowers and trees and vegetables but they do not respect insects.

So let's do that. When I work in my yard the bugs are all over. Ground bees are flying in and out around me and for the most part the mosquitoes don't bother me. I love to sit and watch a bug crawling around on a plant. Insects are so diverse in looks that each one is a design original.

One day I sat in the house near a screened window just watching life evolve in my back yard. The interesting part was that the sun was shining directly on the area close to the house but the area farther away from the house was in shadows. So what I saw looked like dust particles one sometime sees in the air. They were dancing around like gypsies in a musical.

First I watched a couple of large butterflies that were so happy to have found the spearmint patch in full blossom. They flitted from one purple top to another and soon they were joined by a white moth.

As I sat and watched, there were hundreds of small dots of sunlit bugs of all kinds. Some buzzed around while other were just traveling through, looking like a small comet.

Why do people dislike bugs? Is it because they eat some of the plants? Is it because they attack people? Is it because they are attracted to things people have that they consider their food? I guess it could be all those things or why else would they be bugs, bugging humans.

Insects have a job to do, actually many jobs and they work very hard at them. The first job is to pollinate plants so that each plant can become the best that it can be. This of itself is a very big job. Most people think that only bees do this but all insects do it. Some plants don't even flower without insects to help them.

Another job that insects have is recycling what is no longer needed. People don't think about this side of it. They just don't want "Bugs" in their dying food. Why did I put it that way? Because when something is harvested, it is fresh only for a very short time and then it starts to die. It is the job of insects to take care of that. When a bug smells something that has been dead for a long time, he feels badly as maybe he hasn't been doing his job. How about a "meat" sandwich? Now here is an animal that not only died a long time ago but a part of it has been chemical treated to keep it from recycling. To a bug, this needs to be handled.

When my neighbor would work in her yard, the ground bees would bother her. I suggested putting some sugar water in a jar cover and placing it a long way from where she is working. It worked for her.

For me, I just tell them the area that I want to work on and we have no problem. Why is that so? Because everything knows that it is all about co-creating. As it is my garden, then I must do the work to make it look good and produce. Production can be whatever that plant was created to do. It might be flowers. It might be leaves. It might be roots that I plan to harvest.

Each plant has something for us.

There are times when a new plant appears in my yard. I never know what to expect but enjoy all the presents that I am given. I like to find out about the new resident. It is the same with insects. I see someone that I have never met before and want to know who it is and what their job is.

About a block away from my house, the residents of another house had a "bug light" in their back yard. I could hear the hum of this machine all of the time. So I went to check on it. I found that

195

the "bug light" was turned on all day and most of the night while the people of that house had all their windows closed. I could also hear their air-conditioner working. I guess that it was just in case they might decide to come out into their back yard at any time? Even though it was a block away, I put a note in their mail box asking them not to leave the "Bug light" on all the time as I was losing a lot of butterflies, lady bugs and many other beneficial insects.

The thing that I really noticed was the decline in Lightening Bugs in my back yard that year. I love to go outside at night when the Lightening Bugs are flitting all over the place. It is like a fairyland. Now add a few Devas that come out to play after their charges are settled for the night...it is wonderful. What did Shakespeare say about a "midsummer's night...." One can't find a more emotional setting than that.

In case you want to know, there are Devas of insects and we can talk to them. When we had gypsy moths, we were told to find out what the moths needed to stay healthy without overrunning the tree. We did and they never took more leaves than they needed. (It was a very large oak tree)

Gardeners are learning about degree days. This is the number of degrees over 50 degrees Fahrenheit that accumulates as the days warm up in the spring. It seems that scientist have figured out that certain insects "wake up" when there have been say, 80 accumulated degrees of heat above 50 degrees. So in April we have four days that get to be 52 degrees. That is 2 degrees times 4 days and we have 8 accumulated degree days. As you can see this is all very scientific but insects really aren't as reliable as that. I think it would be hard to find the insect that is suppose to come out of hibernation the day one hits 80 degree days or whatever that insect is scheduled at.

At least in the science of gardening, humans recognize the value of insects.

Let's look at a nice neighborhood where there are a lot of pretty houses. When I walk down a street like this or bike past these houses; I find that most of them have little signs on their lawn telling people that it has just been sprayed with a toxin. This means that chemicals were put on the plants in that yard to keep the weeds out and the bugs down.   Does it work? I see these people out there really working on their yards. They don't have any idea how harmful all of the chemicals are and not just to the insects but I am talking about their own health and that of their animals. As an herbalist I have treated dogs who are victims of these sprays.

Tonight I saw a new invention to keep bugs out of your house. It is electronic and gets plugged into the wall. Then a vibration of a certain value is sent into the wiring system of your house. This sounds so great until you stop to think about it. If everything in this world is vibrational, the wood table vibrates at a different rate than the window glass, what vibration do they use on bugs? It is possible that the vibration would damage some cells in a bug? Why is it not going to damage something in me? I am very sensitive to vibrations so I had to asked my husband not to consider getting this gadget.

We are in the middle of a recession /depression and it is a wonderful thing. I know, I have warped values but will people continue to purchase these extras like having the lawn sprayed four times a summer and houses debugged when they aren't sure financially what the future holds? Perhaps all things happen for a reason?

To keep my yard from being over whelmed by insects, I have bird houses all over the place. Even when I was sitting at the windowsill watching the bugs in the sunlight, a wren was sitting on the top of the tomato stake looking at the whole picture from her point of view. To her, she probably saw a banquet.

What is it that they say, "Life is a jungle." We think that means in the office/work place or maybe in the wilderness or woods but the jungle is in our own backyards. If we are really truthful, we will realize that the jungle is right here, inside of us too. We are always trying to find ways to survive and do the right thing.

Appreciate everything around you including the little things/ bugs

Dowsing

On my first trip to Boulder, Colorado to attend classes with Rev. Hanna Kroeger, I met my California-sister Betty at the Denver airport. We took a shuttle to Boulder and checked in at Hanna's retreat. We were assigned a room together on the end of the dormitory. The classes didn't start until the next morning so we spend that evening getting acquainted with the other people who had come from all over the U. S.; we even met a lady that was from Prince Edward Island, Canada.

In the middle of night, I got really sick. I was up and down and in the bathroom a lot. My sister woke up early the next morning and asked how I felt. I told her that I had been sick most of the night. She told me that she was going to talk to Hanna. I really didn't want her to do that because Hanna was probably getting set up to do her class. My sister is as stubborn as I am and she went.

She came back with Hanna who held out a tissue for me, telling me to spit on it. I did that thinking that she was going to put it under a microscope and find out what was wrong with me. She was back in a flash. She has a bottle of Vibrational* Salmonella with her. She looked in the tea cup that I had been drinking out of, and then put 15 drops from this bottle in my tea. She told me to do the same thing in an hourand then she left.

Within a short time my sister left to go to class. I drank what was left of my tea with the drops in it and sat on the bed trying to decide if my stomach was going to settle down or not. About five minutes later, I was starting to feel better. I thought that maybe if I took a shower and climbed into fresh clothes, I would feel much better.

Within twenty minutes, I was feeling really well. I had showered and changed so why was I sitting here? I got my note pad and my pen, then put 15 drops of "that stuff" in water and went to class. I missed out on the introductions to the classes but was there before an hour had past.

What would they have done if I had gone to an emergency room? Well, they might have just let me sit to see how I was doing or if things didn't seem to settle down they could have pumped my stomach and kept me there for observation for the remainder of the morning or maybe the rest of the day.

Later, I found out that Hanna had dowsed to find out what was wrong with me and then gave me what was needed to counteract the problem.

By the end of the first day, she told us to practice dowsing and showed us how to do it. She said that for everyone, it was different. We should ask to be shown our "yes" response and then ask to be shown our "no" response. At first I didn't think I was getting any answers because the pendulum just hung there. What I have since learned is that when it "digs" in and acts like a plum line, that is my NO answer. (A plum line is a weighted line that is being pulled by earth's gravity to hang straight down.) When my pendulum goes in a circle that is my YES answer.

As I have mentioned, each person is different. I know a lady whose pendulum circles clockwise for "yes" and circles counter-clockwise for "no". Another person that I know gets her answers from a swinging pendulum. If it swings out and back, it is her "yes" and if it swings to both sides of her, it is her "No".

This really didn't seem strange to me because I remember my Grandpa using a split willow to find where to drill the wells when we were building our houses. Each of the three spots that he picked brought in an artesian well.

Hanna told us that we could dowse for health. By dowsing, we were accessing things that we had no knowledge of but spirit did. As an example, I don't know if anyone has parasites in their body but by dowsing, I not only can say yes or no but I can actually tell them what kind is there.

We were told the rules of dowsing. If someone asks you to do it, you may but you are not allowed to get information about people that have not given you permission to do this.

Hanna told us that we were using the person's vibrational energy to do this. She would have a person sit by her side as she checked them out with their permission or she said that we could use a saliva sample of that person. By giving a saliva sample, that person was giving permission to be checked and we were allowed to find out what was going on with them health-wise.

She mentioned that we could dowse from a picture of a person too. How did she put this? "You are known by your vibrations." Each of us has a different personal vibration. If we use a picture, it must be one taken since that person's last blood transfusion or transplant as these change the vibrations of a person. A blood transfusion and transplants bring with them the traits of the donor. I also tell people that the picture can't have pets in it, as I don't want to find out that the person has fleas. (Personal joke)

Once someone sent me a picture of a couple and I had to write back to tell them that one of them had problems but I didn't know which one.

Another time I gave a picture back to a lady and told her that I wasn't able to get anything. Either that person has some very strong personal protection and I am not allowed in or I wasn't given permission to check him. She then mentioned that he didn't know anything about this but she was going to surprise him. I don't think so!

Dowsing can be another way to get in touch with the spirit world. When I dowse, I find it very helpful to ask my guardian angels to assist me in helping someone else. I ask for protection from all negative sources. I ask that I be given only the information that would help the person or persons involved to move ahead or heal their bodies.

Sometimes we don't want to look at things that would help us move ahead. Once I dowsed for a lady and couldn't get any information. My answer to that is that she must not want it done or that she has some very strong personal beliefs that hinder this.

She told me that a lot of people have told her this same thing. It could be that she needs to learn about everything on her own.

Hanna talked about reading books with a pendulum. She said that we could ask to be shown the chapters in a book that we need to read to get the essence of that book and then not have to read the whole book. Or we can ask where we should live. Maybe we can ask if this is a good deal for us or if we should think about working here. Sometimes we feel so helpless and unable to move ahead. Dowsing can be helpful.

* Vibrational – Hanna has products that negate different medical problems. We all know that the world is made up of vibrations and in Europe there is a machine that can measure each vibration of something. Example: protozoa, a tiny one celled parasite that can create arthritis in joints. The machines might find that protozoa vibrates at -10, so Hanna puts together a combination that contains a +10. Thus the two cancel each other out and the body will not have this situation to deal with.

A Shaman

What would it be like to be a Shaman, a healer and leader? One has to "know thyself" well. One has to understand what powers are available and how to use them. Most people don't have the slightest idea of just how powerful they really are.

It is my belief that at one time, this was my responsibility. Maybe it still is? As I learned about healing herbs, I know that this is not a new thing for me to learn. I have just gotten reacquainted with one of my talents. Plants and I have been friends for a very long time.

My tribe still brings things to me to be healed. Yesterday one of them was being attacked by something not nice. Herbs aren't the only way to heal. Sometimes we have to listen inside of ourselves to find out which way would be the best way to handle a particular situation. Sometimes the Shaman must use his power to protect the tribe from enemies, seen or unseen. We use what has the most power for the situation. It might be just to block the incoming energy. We are to suggest what would be the best protection in any case.

Moving the energy of the sky to Mother Earth or the other way around is a fun thing to do. Moving Energy is part of the Shaman's job, as is blocking harmful energies.

Doing ceremonies seems to come naturally for me. What I found is that most people do not recognize the power of words. When we speak, we create a vibration that can create wonderful things or destructive things. It is all up to the speaker. Vibrations can last a very long time. I remember when my son told me not to say, "always" and "never" as we don't fully understand the meaning of either of those. These energies sent out waves that continue to travel and some of them are reflected back at us.

It didn't seem at all that strange to do a candlelight service for a favorite Aunt by her grave stone when our family returned from a trip. This is part of the Shaman's job. Saying Good-bye to a wonderful lady like Aunt Ruth was something I felt very good about. Talking about the memories that we all had encompassing each other was a wonderful way to say good-bye. I cannot imagine having my funeral in a building away from nature.

While visiting Sedonia, we went to a medicine wheel. I asked if I could do a blessing with the eucalyptus leaves that I had collected from along the Colorado River. It felt right to give thanks and praise to the four corners of the Earth, to Father Sky and Mother Earth. I don't think we do that enough but then we have been trained to pray to get things instead of giving thanks and praise.

Why do I feel so close to this dimension of my world? How about the time that I watched Dances With Wolves and then for a long time I couldn't stop crying. It was so real to me. I cried as I hauled a blanket outside along with some yarn and some feathers that I had been given. I sat on my blanket and wove the feathers into braids of yarn. Finally I got it just about the way I wanted it so I went into the garage to find a pole. I made a circle of vine, then attached the feathered cords to it and put all of this on the pole. I took it to the P garden and stood this up in the garden. (The P garden was named this as it is anchored by a pear tree and a plum tree.) I asked how to explain it to others and was told that it was a blessing for our property. I watched as the feathers twirled on the ends of their braids. Then I was told to put more blue on it so I hot glued some blue rocks and shells that I had. Then I knew that it was done.

Sometimes the information is just there and sometimes one has to allow it to come. Shamans deal with all kinds of things and whatever works is the right thing.

I have used candles to heal people. Why did the candles work? I have no idea but I felt that candles were needed.

One time I put rocks all over the person to pull out the negativity and ground her. It seemed to work. Some people are open to anything even if they don't understand it. Other people can't handle "different". (Not an unusual thought from most people.)

How I think isn't in line with how most people think. My life doesn't travel in a "normal" direction. I have always felt that I walked a line between two worlds.

Before I learned about power, I had the opportunity to learn what I was capable of controlling. I found the most people are not aware of how much they are controlled. This is a planet of free choice and it was designed that way for a reason. The first rule is to allow each being the ability to make choices, right or wrong. Even assisting them in making the choice must be done by pointing out or helping them to see all the different options that they have.

What kind of magical powers do we have? We have a lot of power if we aren't afraid to use it. One of my mentors told me that the beings in bodies are more powerful than the beings without bodies. I have used that information a few times. We have been empowered with intuitive brains that are ready to tell us what we need to know. Our "librarian" has so much information that can be accessed for any occasion. So why don't most people know about this, because they are so afraid of looking different.

When one walks in many worlds, they seem to be different from those around them, but in truth they aren't because there is only one world. We all live here even the unseen live here. May I always use my power for the greatest good!

Ɖanna's Ϲⅅagic

Tonight I have been remembering a wonderful wizard that I met in 1992. She came into my life with all the spunk that a 4 foot 6 person can. She stood 10 feet tall in ideas, some of which were beyond belief. By now most of you know that I am talking about Reverend Hanna Kroeger of Boulder Colorado.

What first attracted me to her was that she seemed to have answers to things that I hadn't even thought about before. At the time I had just gotten custody of my mother who had a form of Alzheimer's disease and I was looking for answers.

While reminiscing tonight I remembered some of the things that I watched this lady do. She would put her right hand above a reclined persons head and the left hand below their tail bone, never touching the body in order to release blood clots that were in that body. And to stop bleeding she would do the opposite, with the left hand over the head and the right hand under the tailbone. I remember when she told about the service man that came back from Vietnam and he was telling her that this method saved many men over there.

Such a simple thing yet Hanna was full of these simple things that one could do that were "magic" to most of us.

How about putting one's right hand on a forehead and the left hand at the back-base of the head for pneumonia. Who would even think that it would work? She told us to leave our hands there until the person takes a very deep breath.

She was full of this kind of information. I remember when she told us that people with a vitamin deficiency have more problems early in the morning but a person with mineral deficiency will have their problems in the evening. Maybe someone reading this will be able to figure out which of the two is their problem?

One class that she gave was about Vitamins. She said that Vitamin A is manufactured in the right collar bone. Vitamin B-12 is manufactured in the left collar bone. Vitamin D is manufactured in the sternum. Vitamin E is manufactured in the long ribs. Finally she said that Vitamin P feeds the brain and capillaries, this is Bioflavonoids and they are found in food pigments.

Hanna mentioned that we need to know what is happening in our bodies. If one pushes up on the bottom of our cheek bone and it hurts, we have a bacterial infection somewhere .

Every time I would turn around she was telling us or showing us something amazing. One time she checked out a student in our group and found that his left scapula (The bone attached to the top of the arm, sitting on the back) was lower than the right one. With a wooden pencil, a hammer and a bones chart of the human body; she adjusted his bones. She put the erasure of the pencil on the bone to be moved and had the student sit next to the chart touching it, then she pounded the pencil with a hammer until she saw the student's bone in the right place. It really worked.

She taught us how to dowse and told us that we could use this method to find water, even ask how deep it would be and if it was worth digging a well here. She told us that we would get overwhelmed with books to read so we could dowse to find out which chapters to read to get the essence of the book. And regarding maps, the question to ask is "where does God want me to be?" She mentioned that we are always within 300 yards of help. Now that help might just be a log to get under until the storm is over.

Hanna was very strong on personal protection. Her instructions were to put your protection vibration on things. To do this one can brush a hand over the book, picture, check and no one can influence it. She mentioned that when someone is being a bother, we pound our right fist into our left palm twice and say, "What in God's name are you doing here?" She mentioned that this works for an IRS check up and they won't find anything wrong.

I have a personal belief that our legal system is very flawed. No one is given enough information to make a good decision. I would need a whole lot more just to give a decision to my children on anything. But we are asked to decide things that affect people's lives forever. Therefore when I get jury duty notice, I use the "What in God's name are you doing to me?" Usually the court cases that I am called to gets settled out of court.

Hanna was so spunky and knowledgeable. When she lived in Germany she was a nurse and apparently a very good one because she mentioned that the doctors would have her close when she attended them in surgery.

She had a forgiveness formula. It was her contention that one should write it all out at night before going to bed and in the morning read what one wrote, then burn it. She said to do this until one doesn't have anything to write and suggests that it should be gone in 7 days. Once she mentioned that when we write our problems out they get smaller but when we talk them out, they get bigger.

One time when she was walking through the dining hall, she stopped by someone who had a slice of bread. She told them to tear the bread and bless it. This staff of life had been baked and then its life was sliced with a knife so it needed to be torn and blessed. Rolls don't need to this, as they don't get cut with a weapon.

Mint was the subject of one of her talks. She said that it brings you to the "Vau" condition. With her accent, I thought she meant "Wow" but she didn't. She showed us in the Bible that "Vau" raises you closer to the God level. With regard to mint, she suggested putting a sprig of peppermint on the picture of someone having surgery to help them heal faster.

At the time that I was hearing all of this, it was a different language for me. This little wizard had so many things that I couldn't believe them all. (That didn't mean that I didn't write them down.) It has taken me a long time to make some of these a reality in my life.

One day she pulled me aside and told me that she wanted to show me something. (Why me?) We walked to the door of her apartment and she told me to wait there. Soon she came back with a photo album of pictures. She opened the book up and showed me a picture that was covered with grey smoke. All I could see in the picture was the bottom part of a wheel that might have been a wheel chair. She told me that this person was loaded with evil spirits and after she worked on him, he could walk.

Then she showed me a lady in a picture holding hands with a small child on each side of her. I couldn't see her face very well as a white cloudy circle was in the way. Hanna told me that this lady was very verbally abusive and her language was that of a sailor. After working with her, she became a very sweet person.

I asked Hanna how she got these pictures with evil spirits showing in them. She said that she used to have a little black box and she would put the pictures in the box for a while, when they came out she could see the cloudiness of evil. She then looked at me and told me that the government came to her place one time and that they took the black box. I told her that I hoped she made another one; she smiled with the biggest smirk while closing her book then left to put it away. What a magician!

Hanna mentioned that Silver protects us from evil as the dark forces can't get through silver. When I learned that I started to wear silver on my person.

With regard to silver, she taught us not to use chemical cleaners on our silverware but to clean it with salt and baking soda. Her other advice was to use our silverware and let the children inherit the stainless steel. As a nurse in Germany, there was a box of silver spoons and the babies and very elderly were fed with sterling cutlery. It seems that silver is very antibiotic.

She mentioned a couple of interesting things that I wish to pass along. The first one is that people who can't taste things have a lack of Zinc in their systems. Zinc is found in Spinach, Cucumbers, Black Beans, Plums, Asparagus, Tomatoes, Cauliflower, Brussels sprouts and nuts of all kinds.

The other loss is the loss of smell. My Aunt Milly had this and Hanna said that it is Cadmium poisoning. She has a remedy to get the Cadmium out of the body. How does one get it? It comes in with colored material. We have this wonderful purple shirt and as we sweat it pulls the dye out and allows it to be absorbed into our bodies. (The sweat and the dye make a tincture and the skin takes it in.)

When it came to the brain, she talked about sesame seed as building strong minded people. She also talked a lot about crystals. They are thought enhancers. They magnify our thoughts.

(At one time they were used to enhance radio reception) So when I dowse, I never use a crystal pendulum as I don't want my ideas out there, I want to know what is really so.

She worked with herbs but then she worked with everything. What she liked about herbs was the fact that they didn't drive chemicals into the system.

She talked about how powerful the spoken word was. It was her idea that when the body has a problem, one can tell it to go away. She said that "A single voice is most powerful. Words and songs are very powerful." In one session she had us all put our hands on a cancer person and shout , "SHU, SHU, SHU. "

I find that the song from the Sound of Music with the entire scale is a wonderful one to use as it hits all the notes. What I do is hum with my teeth almost closed. The vibration in the teeth is felt through the whole skeleton as they are all connected.

I had a virus one time and the doctor did a punch biopsy. The test came back saying it was a virus but the area cleaned itself up. The doctor told me that this happens sometimes when an area is disturbed. I guess my humming could do the disturbing. We have talked about vibrations in other stories in this book.

I really admired this little lady. Hanna would tell it like it was. Her two main books are GOD HELPS THOSE WHO HELP THEMSELVES and THE SEVEN SPIRITUAL CAUSES OF ILL HEALTH. She taught us how to use these two books to help those around us.

A lot of interesting people have come into my life but this wonderful little wizard of a woman changed the direction of mine for good.

Little Beings

In the reading that I have done over the years, I learned that animals have the ability to take on our physical problems, thus helping us to live longer and better. They are truly here to help us and perhaps that is why a lot of animals are being allowed into nursing homes at this time?

One set of books, (Sorry I don't remember the reference) was about a bed-bound man who had two cats. I believe he lived in Canada and it was supposed to be a true story. He used to send his cats shopping for him. They would come back and show him their pictures and he knew what store handled what he was looking for and could order it.

There have been few years in my life when I have been without a pet. How about the dog that sat patiently next to me on the back steps when I was feeling really down, then with those trusting eyes, told me it was going to be better soon. They never scold or give advice on what should have been done. They are just there. Isn't it nice to have a friend that doesn't judge?

I do have to mention that I had a cat named lady who would come up on my lap if I was crying about something and swat me in the face. That always made me laugh. I guess she knew that it would. What a treasure. She was a bossy cat who was raised with a dog and when that dog died, she took over and learned how to growl at strangers. Then we got a companion cat for her, she let the new cat know just whose house this was.

I have pictures of all the animals that we have had in the last 35 years. I even did a watercolor painting of one of them and gave it to the breeder who didn't charge me for her. I even did a charcoal drawing of the dog we had that our son Blaine helped to train.

Animals and Blaine just go together. He took me to Bay Park in Green Bay and showed me a wolf that lives there with a pack of other wolves. This one recognizes him and comes to the fence when he arrives. Blaine usually had a hunk of jerky in his pocket for this one.

One time Blaine took me to a pet store and introduced me to a large bird. Blaine petted her and talked to her. Then he told me to pet her. She bit me. I think she thought I was a rival.

This bird will probably out live me. I like to remember that a lot of animals do have shorter lives than humans even if some live for a very long time, like this bird. When my cat wants attention, I can spare time in my life to give her attention.

Blaine has slept in our dog house because he didn't want his dog to be alone. He always trains them and they mind him. Last week he was here and Snowy came up to greet him. He leaned down, petted and talked to her. She followed him around the whole time he was here. She even licked him to let him know that she liked his vibrations.

Some people are able to put out a vibration of caring about those around them. Animals as well as other people seem to sense this and gravitate to these people. I am not sure if people understand the importance of this.

Each animal wants to help humans but we are very barbarous as a species so that the vibration that usually preceding us is one of anger or supremacy or even hurtful power. Animals are so sensitive that they pick up on this right away and get out of our way.

As humans, we used to have this ability to sense danger before we got in the middle of it but now only our animals can do this. Today as I was walking home from downtown, a dog barked pleasantly from the garage of one of the buildings that I went by. I acknowledged him and told him that he was doing a very good job. You see, when I have gone by there before, small children are playing in the driveway or yard and today was no exception. The kids were on the play equipment and this dog just wanted everyone to know that he was on duty as there wasn't an adult around.

The animals on this planet want to be of service to humans. In a book that I recently read, the main character lives in a wooded area and the animals provide her with food and not in the way we think. They do not give their lives for her but instead bring her food in the form of nuts and berries and anything that would be helpful. I even read where a small rodent chewed the food up and then put it into the mouth of her human child who was crying, thinking that he was hungry. This sounds more like fiction than fact but I have been assured that it is factual.

Knowing that all plants and animals on this planet have a spiritual being or Deva that is there to help them, I get upset when someone tells me, "Well, they are just animals." For that matter, so are we, just animals.

I was talking to a lady once and in the conversation I mentioned something about being " a meat body or something about our meat bodies..." She got really upset and told me that she wasn't a meat body. I apologized and told her that we really are meat bodies that house a spiritual being. Am not sure how she took that but maybe it was the first time she ever looked at life like that?

It is time for humans to wake up and understand the world around us is made up of many different beings, and we are just one of the many. Little beings are important in our world. Remember that the next time you encounter one.

Planet of Choice

After reading this book up to this point, one would think that the author is the luckiest person in the world. Well, I am, but not in the way that you think. One might think, *Gee she can get answers to all her questions and when a problem pops up, there are always answers for her.*

This is not so.

We are on this planet to learn. How can we learn if someone else is handling all our problems? In this book I have tried to show you how to find some of your own answers. Everyone has dark days, but that shouldn't send us on a chemical trip; these are just the times when one doesn't know what step to take next.

Life is good as it gives us many choices for each problem.

Recently I was acting as a sounding board for a friend of mine. He was trying to figure out what he should do regarding his present-time problem. I listened to him and helped him dig out all of his options; if there weren't options toward a solution, he wouldn't have a problem.

When we are confronted with something that isn't working, we are only looking at one side of this situation and usually with it right in our faces. There are 6 sides to a box and by sharing only one side with someone, they might be able to see the sides of it that you can't. If a Box is sitting on the floor, you are able to see three sides of it from your vantage point but the person on the other side of the box sees the sides that you don't.

Now which of these options *felt* (there is that word again) the best to him? I have even dowsed for him to help him get assistance on which solution might be better than others. Still, I can't make the decision for him.

I have a quote on my refrigerator that my son left there. "Now, as we look over problems and solutions, we discover that an individual's brightness depends upon his ability to arrive at solutions. But his sanity depends on his ability to invent problems. Got that? A great oddity." LRH

One time my daughter got a D in one of her subjects and she said something that has followed me all through life. She said, "They never gave me credit for what I did learn." I guess they expected her to learn what they wanted her to learn.

I heard the same thing put in a different way last week. A salesman said, "I do make mistakes but I learn so much from them."

When I am working on a watercolor painting and something strange happens to the paint... maybe it runs into a place that I didn't want it to, I find that it turns out even better than I had planned. I have used places like this to make water drops sitting on the leaf or a rock that I wouldn't have put there but really belongs there.

Our mistakes make us human.

Every choice that we make takes us into our future. Most of us know that we create our futures by our todays.

What if we are being judgmental instead of being open to what is happening in front of us? When I went through that lesson, the repercussions came back at me within 24 hours; sort of like "getting hit on the head" spiritual training. How many times have you said," Right!" knowing that what you just did wasn't right at all but at that moment it seemed to be. Looking back you say something like, *"Well, I learned something that time."*

One article in this book talks about how strong the WORD is. What we say and even what we *think* is powerful and helps create the world that we live in.

Hanna Kroeger, my mentor, talked a lot about vibrations and even introduced a line of vibrational medicines. I prefer them to homoeopathy because they do not contain any of the substance for which they are to be used. One of my friends took this vibrational concept further. She writes the name of the problem; let's say "Shingles" on a piece of paper then puts a circle around it and a diagonal line through the circle; meaning "no Shingles". She then carries this on her person to create the vibration of no shingles in that body. I have even known where she attaches a WORD to her dog's collar for him to wear.

Recently a friend of mine called to tell me that she was in the process of passing a kidney stone and had bloody urine. I suggested that she write Hydrangea on a piece of paper and carry it on her person. Hydrangea root will dissolve stones in the body. By putting this vibration around her, she was able to eliminate it. I also suggest adding vinegar to her drinking water. She told me next day that within two hours of carrying the paper with the word "Hydrangea" on it, her urine wasn't bloody anymore and that she was going to start the vinegar.

I wish to talk about pledges and promises now. How powerful is the word? As a young girl, I went with my boyfriend to his church late at night. We turn on lights at the altar and we made pledges and promises to each other there in front of God. These are still active even though more than 50 years have gone by and we have both moved on in our lives. We are still connected with the words that were spoken. Neither of us understood what we were doing at that time.

We speak words whose meanings and power are not fully understood and find these words are controlling our lives to a degree. Most people do not know how to rescind any of these and it limits what we do in the future. As a planet of choice, we have the ability to choose to move these blocks out of our way. Moving blocks of promises or pledges is not something that we have ever been taught how to do or even that it is possible.

This is a planet of choice and we have many choices. Most of us have never been introduced to a lot of our choices.

My son told me, "Mom, don't use the words "Never" or "Always" or "Forever". They lock us into a very narrow choice pattern on this planet. " He is right.

215

How about the person that gives away everything they have to the point of not having enough to live on? Perhaps they made a pledge of poverty somewhere in their past and it is impinging on the choices that they can make in present-time.

How about giving a pledge of loyalty to a group and later finding flaws in the group so one needs to leave; does the pledge dissipate?

We are allowed to make choices and each one should be made based on the best solution for every situation but that doesn't always happen. It is at this time that we send up the plea, "Why me God"? What can we do then? My daughter tells me that an "attitude adjustment" is called for in those times. As we adjust to the new situation, we will find answers coming to us. I know you think that because I never walk alone that I don't have to make choices, but I do. The difference is that if we adjust out thinking, we will see that what looked like a problem is just a stepping stone in another direction of life.

Each choice that one makes creates his or her reality. I call them 90 degree turns as I can travel along in life and hit a wall. The next thing I know, I am doing something completely different.

When I look back at all the decisions that I have had to make, I find that they have made me the person that I presently am. This is part of the learning process that we are here for. Do I want to make more choices? Yes. This adventure called life is ongoing. What is the saying, "Enjoy the ride" and make some wonderful choices.

In this book I have given you many choices to choose from; some of the information is about using medicinal plants, some are about the connection we have with the spiritual realm. All are ways to heal our bodies and our infinite beings. It doesn't make any difference what you chose because this is a planet of choices.

I have been told that Life is a game. It has players, a playing field, choices, restrictions, rewards and penalties. It's your move!

Leap of Faith

When we learn about herbs and all the great things that they are capable of helping us with, we are still intimidated about using them because we have not been trained to do this. Our training tells us that only doctors or nurses can help us.

With this in mind, I find that every time I give a person a leaf to chew on, they hold it in their hands like I have just handed them poison. So unless I put a leaf from that same plant into my mouth, this person will just study the leaf. It could be a Peppermint leaf or a Stevia leaf, what it is doesn't really matter except that it is not found in the produce section of the local grocery store.

I have to admit that I am also in this category when it comes to harvesting mushrooms. Unless I was with someone who has done this before and lived to tell the story, I would feel the same way.

So the reader of this book is really taking a leap of faith by deciding that these things really might work. I am always amazed at how a plant is able to do all the things that I have learned about each and every one of them. The thing is that they really do them.

Probably the first thing a reader might want to do is learn to identify the plants that live in their local area. Books are really helpful but sometimes it is nice to find the person that already can identify them. An herb walk is nice with a knowledgeable herbalist. Botanical gardens are wonderful where the plants are labeled so we can study each plant before using it. I find books that have drawings in them are most helpful. Photos tend to blur the outlines of the leaves or leave out the most important part of the plant.

For those of you who just want to use herbs and do not want to harvest them yourselves, Health food stores that carry bulk herbs or even capsules are a nice comfortable place to be. For the most part, one can rely on what the label says.

It always amazes me to find that a person will down two or three different kinds of pills that he picked up at Walgreens but when confronted with an herbal combination that does the very same thing without any side effects, they tend to distrust it.

Once something has been used successfully, like Dr. Christopher's herbal combination for sinus congestion, they will no longer go to Walgreens for some over-the-counter decongestant.

It is with a leap of faith that we all learn new things. May you have found what you needed to make this leap, somewhere in this book.

Resources - Part Two

Buhner, Stephen Harrod, **The Lost Language Of Plants,** Chelsea Green Publishing, White River Junction, VT., 2002

Carson, Rachel, **Silent Spring,** Houghton Mifflin Co, Boston, Ma. 1962

Eno, Paul F., **Turning Home,** New River Press, Woonsocket, RI, 2006

Gurudas, **The Spiritual Properties Of Herbs,** Cassandra Press, San Rafael, CA. 1988

Hawken, Paul, **The Magic Of Findhorn,** Harper and Row, New York, 1975

Hoffmann, Wendell H., **Using Energy To Heal,** Printed in the US of A, 1979, Revised and Updated 1992

Kelly, Penny, **Robes – A Book Of Coming Changes**, Authors Choice Press, New York, 1999

Kelly, Penny, **The Elves Of Lily Hill Farm – A Partnership With Nature**, Authors Choice press, New York,1997

Kroeger, Hanna Rev., **God Helps Those That Help Themselves,** copyrighted 1984

Kroeger, Hanna Rev., **The Seven Spiritual Causes of Ill Health.,** copyrighted 1988

Maclean, Dorothy, **To Honor The Earth,** HarperCollins Publisher, NY., 1991

Megre, Vladimir, **Anastasia,** Ringing Cedars Press, HI.,2005

Roads, Michael J. **Talking With Nature,** H.J. Kramer, Tiburon, CA. 1985

Tompkins, Peter & Bird, Christopher, **The Secret Life Of Plants,** Harper and Row, Publishers, New York, NY. 1973

Wright, Machaelle Small, **Behaving As If The God In All Life Mattered,** Perelandra, Ltd., Warrenton, VA. 1997